Tai Chi for Weight Loss

The Complete Exercise Guide for Seniors and Beginners to Burn Fat, Increase Strength, and Feel Younger — 28-Day Workout Program, 10 Mins a Day, No Gym Needed

Jing Weston

Disclaimer

This book is intended for general informational and educational purposes only. The exercises and guidance contained in this publication are not a substitute for professional medical advice, diagnosis, or treatment. Always consult your physician or qualified healthcare provider before beginning any new exercise program, particularly if you have a pre-existing medical condition, recent injury, or surgery.

The author and publisher assume no responsibility for any injury, loss, or damage incurred as a result of the use or application of information contained in this book.

Table of Contents

A Note from the Author

There is a particular kind of frustration that comes after sixty. Not the frustration of failure, exactly. More the frustration of surprise. You do what you have always done, eat more or less how you have always eaten, try to stay active, and the body does not respond the way it used to. The weight sits differently. The joints take longer to warm up. The energy that was always just there, ready when you needed it, now has to be coaxed.

I have watched this happen with hundreds of people over the years. Men and women who were active most of their lives, who walked dogs and gardened and worked physical jobs, suddenly finding that the rules had changed without anyone telling them. The advice they got, more exercise, fewer calories, push harder, was the same advice that had worked at forty and did not work anymore. That gap, between what they were being told and what was actually happening in their bodies, was where most of them gave up.

I came to Tai Chi through an injury. I was in my early forties, dealing with a knee that had decided it was done with impact, and someone suggested I try a class. I went reluctantly. I left curious. Within a few months I had stopped tolerating something and started practicing something. The knee improved. The sleep improved. Something in the quality of how I moved through a day changed in a way that was hard to name but easy to feel.

That was more than twenty years ago. Since then I have worked with older adults in group settings and one-on-one. People who came in with bad hips and worse morale. People who had been told to exercise and had no idea where to start. People who were skeptical and tired and willing to give one more thing a try. What I can tell you from all of that time is this: the body does not stop responding. It slows down. It changes what it responds to. But it does not stop.

Tai Chi works for older adults for reasons that are not obvious at first. It is not simply that it is gentle. Gentle alone does not change a body. Tai Chi works because it combines controlled sustained movement with breath coordination and mental focus in a way that targets the exact mechanisms that determine how a body ages: cortisol regulation, muscle preservation, joint lubrication, balance. It does not burn calories the way a spin class does. It does something more useful at this stage of life. I explain exactly what that is in the chapters ahead.

This book is a 28-day program, and the program works. Ten minutes a day is enough to get started. You do not need a gym or special equipment or any previous experience with Tai Chi. What you need is a willingness to show up for yourself each day and follow the steps as they are given.

I want to be honest with you about what to expect. You are not going to lose thirty pounds in a month. Nobody will promise you that here. What you will start to notice, often within the first week, is something quieter. The mornings feel different. The stiffness loosens more quickly. You stand up from a chair and it does not require the same effort. These are not small things. These are the signs that your body is responding.

Read the book through once before you begin the program if you can. The chapters on how Tai Chi affects the body, and the chapter on getting ready, will help you practice with more awareness and get more from the sessions. But if you are the kind of person who needs to start doing before you can settle into reading, go to Chapter Three first, then Chapter Four, then begin Day 1.

Whatever brought you here, I am glad you came. The practice is waiting.

Jing Weston

Before You Begin

Before you take a single step, there are a few things worth settling. They will not take long. But getting them right will make the practice work better from the start.

Medical Disclaimer

Please talk to your doctor before beginning this program. I know that sounds like the standard thing everyone writes at the front of a fitness book, and you have probably read it before and moved past it. I would ask you to take it seriously here.

Tai Chi is among the safest forms of movement available to older adults. The research supports this clearly. But safe does not mean no consideration required. If you have a heart condition, a history of stroke, severe osteoporosis, serious balance issues, or a recent surgery, your doctor needs to know you are starting a movement practice. Not to stop you. To advise you. There is a difference, and a good doctor will help you modify where needed rather than simply say no.

The movements in this book are low-impact. The program is designed for beginners. Every exercise includes a seated option. Still, you know your body and your medical history better than any book can. If something hurts in a way that does not feel like normal effort, stop. Rest. Try again tomorrow or consult someone who can look at you directly. Pain is information. Listen to it.

This book does not treat, cure, or diagnose any medical condition. It is a movement practice guide written for educational purposes. The author and publisher accept no liability for any injury or adverse outcome. Your health decisions are your own.

What You Need

One of the genuine pleasures of Tai Chi is how little it asks of you in terms of equipment. Here is what you actually need.

A clear floor space roughly six feet by four feet. You need room to extend both arms fully to each side and step forward and back without hitting furniture. A living room with the coffee table moved is plenty. The floor should be non-slip and flat.

A sturdy chair without arms. This is for the seated modifications included with every movement. A dining chair is ideal. It should not roll or rock. You will sit toward the front of the seat, so the back of the chair is mostly for reference and occasional balance support.

Comfortable clothing that allows free movement. Loose trousers and a cotton top work well. Nothing that restricts at the shoulders or hips.

Flat shoes or bare feet. Running shoes with thick cushioned soles reduce the ground feedback that Tai Chi depends on. Flat canvas shoes, thin-soled slippers, or bare feet on a non-slip surface are all fine. If you have foot conditions that require specific footwear, wear what your doctor has prescribed.

A quiet space, if possible. Background noise is manageable, but the first few weeks of learning movements benefit from an environment where you can concentrate.

That is the full list. No mat, no weights, no resistance bands, no apps, no downloads. If you have all of the above, you have everything this program requires.

How to Use This Book

This book follows a clear two-track structure, and understanding it will help you get the most from the program.

Chapters One and Two are the foundation. They explain why the body responds the way it does to exercise after sixty, what Tai Chi actually does to change that, and why the science behind slow controlled movement is more relevant to weight loss at this stage than anything involving a treadmill. You do not have to read these chapters before starting the program. But if you understand why a practice works, you tend to do it with more purpose and stay with it longer.

Chapter Three prepares you to practice. It covers posture, breathing, the warm-up sequence you will use before every session, and what to do on the days your body is not cooperating. Read this chapter before Day 1.

Chapter Four is the movement library. All seven Foundation Forms are written out here in full, with step-by-step instructions, breathing cues, and seated modifications. When the 28-day program in Chapter Five tells you to perform a specific movement, this is where you come for the full instructions.

Chapter Five is the 28-day program itself. This is the working heart of the book. You can open it each morning and follow the day's session. Each day tells you exactly what to do and for how long.

Chapters Six through Eight are the support system. Nutrition guidance that does not involve a diet plan. Strength maintenance between sessions. What to do when the 28 days are finished. These chapters extend the value of the practice well beyond the program's end.

If you want to start immediately, go to Chapter Three now, read through the movements in Chapter Four, and return to begin Day 1. If you want the full picture first, read straight through from the beginning. Either approach works.

Chapter 1

Why Your Body Isn't Broken

Something that gets said often to people over sixty, usually with good intentions, is that they need to listen to their body. The problem is that when you have been listening to your body for six decades and it keeps telling you things you were not expecting, the listening starts to feel like bad news.

None of it means your body is broken. It means your body has changed, and the strategies you have been using have not kept up. There is a significant difference, and understanding that difference is the first thing worth doing.

What's Actually Changed After 60

The physiological shifts that happen after sixty are real, measurable, and well-documented. They are not a moral failure. They are biology, and they respond to specific, targeted approaches. Here is what has actually changed.

Muscle mass.

From roughly age thirty, the body begins losing muscle tissue at a rate of about three to five percent per decade without active effort to maintain it. After sixty, that rate accelerates. Less muscle means a lower resting metabolic rate, which means the body burns fewer calories at rest. It also means less structural support around the joints, reduced balance, and reduced capacity to recover from physical effort. This shows up in how you feel getting out of bed in the morning.

The loss is not uniform across the body. The muscles of the legs and core tend to decline faster than those of the upper body, which is one reason why standing up from a low chair, climbing stairs, or walking on uneven ground begins to feel different after sixty. These are the muscles Tai Chi targets most directly, through the sustained soft-bend position that runs through every form.

Metabolic rate.

Even independent of muscle loss, metabolism slows with age due to hormonal changes, reduced mitochondrial efficiency, and changes in how the body processes glucose. The same meal that maintained your weight at forty-five may contribute to weight gain at sixty-five. This is not because you have done something wrong. It is because the body's energy systems work differently now.

The mitochondria, the structures inside cells that convert fuel to energy, become less numerous and less efficient with age. The body produces fewer of them and does not replace damaged ones as quickly. This is one of the reasons older adults often report feeling less energetic even when sleep and nutrition have not changed. Sustained aerobic activity, including the kind of low-intensity sustained movement Tai Chi provides, is one of the few interventions that directly stimulates mitochondrial renewal.

Hormone shifts.

In women, the drop in estrogen after menopause changes where the body stores fat, moving it from the hips and thighs toward the abdomen. In men, declining testosterone reduces the ease of building and maintaining muscle. Both changes affect energy levels, sleep quality, and the body's response to exercise. These shifts do not reverse fully, but they respond to consistent appropriate movement.

Both estrogen and testosterone also influence mood, cognitive sharpness, and the quality of sleep. Their decline is one of the reasons why the post-sixty decade can feel qualitatively different in ways that are hard to attribute to any single cause. What can be said clearly is that exercise, particularly the kind that lowers cortisol and supports sleep, interacts positively with the hormonal environment at this stage in ways that more aggressive approaches do not.

Joint changes.

Cartilage thins with age. Synovial fluid, the lubricant that keeps joints moving smoothly, decreases in production. This is why many people over sixty experience stiffness that was not there before, particularly in the knees, hips, and lower back. High-impact exercise can accelerate this wear. Low-impact flowing movement, the kind Tai Chi provides, actually stimulates synovial fluid production, which is one reason many practitioners report that joints feel better, not worse, after regular practice.

Synovial fluid is not produced passively. It is released in response to movement, particularly slow deliberate movement through the joint's comfortable range. Joints that are not moved regularly produce less fluid and become progressively stiffer. This is the mechanism behind the morning stiffness that most people over sixty recognize: hours of lying still reduces synovial fluid circulation, and the first movements of the day are uncomfortable until the fluid redistributes. Ten minutes of Tai Chi practice, done consistently, meaningfully changes this baseline.

The cortisol response.

The body's cortisol response changes with age. Cortisol, the primary stress hormone, takes longer to return to baseline after a stressful event. Chronically elevated cortisol is one of the main drivers of abdominal fat accumulation in older adults and one of the most underappreciated factors in why traditional weight loss approaches stop working. Chapter Two addresses this in full.

None of this is a list of problems to overcome. It is a description of the terrain. Once you understand the terrain, you can navigate it. Tai Chi addresses most of these changes directly, which is why each of the four sub-sections above has a corresponding solution in the chapters ahead. The physiology is not the problem. The mismatch between that physiology and the standard advice being given to older adults is the problem. This book addresses that mismatch.

Why Traditional Exercise Often Backfires

The well-meaning advice that gets handed to people over sixty, get more exercise, walk every day, try the gym, is not wrong in principle. Movement is medicine. The problem is the type of movement being prescribed and the population it is prescribed for.

High-impact cardio, jogging, aerobics classes, certain group fitness formats, places excessive load on joints that have already lost some of their cushioning. For a forty-year-old with healthy knees and good recovery capacity, this load is manageable. For a sixty-five-year-old with thinning cartilage and a slower recovery cycle, it often produces inflammation, pain, and discouragement. The person does everything right, signs up, shows up, pushes through, and ends up with a sore knee and less motivation than when they started.

The recovery problem is as significant as the impact problem. After sixty, the body takes longer to recover from strenuous exercise. Muscle soreness that resolves in 24 hours at forty may take 48 to 72 hours at sixty-five. If the program calls for three sessions per week and recovery takes three days, the person is never fully recovered before the next session. The cumulative fatigue builds. Motivation drops. The program ends not because the person lacked discipline, but because the program was not designed for their physiology.

Weight training, when poorly programmed, carries similar risks. Lifting heavy loads without proper technique and recovery time can cause joint strain and muscle tears in older adults whose connective tissue is less resilient. This does not mean weight training is off the table. It means it needs to be approached carefully, with appropriate loads and adequate recovery. Most generic gym programs are not designed with this in mind.

Perhaps the most overlooked failure mode of intense exercise for older adults is the cortisol effect. High-intensity exercise, particularly when performed by someone whose body is already under stress from poor sleep, life demands, or chronic inflammation, causes a significant cortisol spike. In younger adults, this spike recovers quickly. In older adults, the elevated cortisol can persist for hours, suppressing fat-burning hormones, disrupting sleep, and contributing to the very abdominal fat the person was trying to lose.

It is possible, in short, to exercise in a way that makes fat loss harder rather than easier. The phrase 'no pain, no gain' was never entirely true. After sixty, it is particularly unhelpful. What the body needs at this stage is consistent intelligent stimulation: movement that lubricates joints rather than grinding them, that builds muscle without provoking injury, and that reduces cortisol rather than spiking it. Tai Chi delivers all three.

What Tai Chi Does That Nothing Else Can

Tai Chi is an ancient Chinese martial art that, in its modern form, is practiced primarily as a movement and wellness system. The version taught in this book is drawn from simplified Yang-style Tai Chi, which is the form most commonly taught to older adults and beginners worldwide because of its gentle pace, clear postures, and documented health benefits. Yang-style was specifically developed with accessibility in mind, and its adoption in clinical settings and senior care programs worldwide reflects a consensus among practitioners and researchers that it is the appropriate form for people beginning later in life.

What makes Tai Chi distinctive is its combination of elements. No other widely practiced exercise form brings together slow controlled full-body movement, coordinated breath, mental focus, and low mechanical load in quite the same way. Each element contributes something the others cannot fully supply on their own. And unlike most exercise systems, the elements reinforce each other: the breathing makes the movement more effective, the movement makes the breathing more natural, and the mental focus makes both more precise. The practice is internally coherent in a way that produces effects greater than any one element would produce in isolation.

The slow controlled movement.

Moving slowly through a posture requires sustained muscle engagement that builds strength without the impact risk of faster movement. Holding a slightly bent knee position while shifting weight from one foot to the other activates the large muscles of the legs, the core, and the stabilizers around the hip in a way that is both effective and safe. The muscles work. The joints are not stressed.

Slow movement also provides continuous proprioceptive challenge. Every small shift of weight requires the nervous system to recalibrate balance. Done daily, this steady low-level challenge rebuilds the neural pathways that control balance and make falls less likely. It is training the nervous system, not just the muscles.

The breath coordination.

Tai Chi uses diaphragmatic breathing throughout practice: deep belly-expanding breaths that activate the parasympathetic nervous system, the body's rest-and-digest state. Regular activation of the parasympathetic system lowers resting cortisol, reduces chronic inflammation, and improves sleep quality. For an older adult whose weight is being driven partly by cortisol and partly by poor sleep, bringing the nervous system into a calmer state through daily practice is a direct intervention, not a side effect.

The mental focus.

Tai Chi requires the practitioner to track where each limb is, how the weight is distributed, and what the breath is doing, all simultaneously. This active mental engagement appears to have its own benefits for cognitive health, and many practitioners report that their practice session is the clearest, quietest part of the day. The focus demanded by the forms is not incidental. It is one of the mechanisms by which the practice works.

Balance improvement.

Multiple published clinical trials have found that regular Tai Chi practice significantly reduces fall risk in older adults. The mechanism is improved proprioception, the body's internal sense of its own position in space, and strengthened stabilizer muscles that respond more quickly when balance is challenged. For older adults, a fall is not a minor inconvenience. It can mean a fracture, a hospital stay, and a long recovery that sets back everything else. Reducing fall risk is not a secondary benefit. It is one of the most important things a practice can offer.

The balance improvements from Tai Chi are not merely about preventing dramatic falls. They show up in smaller, daily ways first: less hesitation when reaching for something, more steadiness when turning quickly, more confidence on uneven surfaces. People who have been avoiding certain situations because of balance uncertainty, stepping off a curb, walking on grass, navigating a crowded space, often find these situations become less fraught within a few weeks of consistent practice. That return of confidence is as real as any measurable balance test result.

The Honest Truth About Fat Loss at This Stage

Fat loss after sixty is slower than it was at thirty. It is slower than the magazines suggest it should be. It is slower than you probably want it to be. That is the truth, and you deserve to hear it directly rather than be managed with optimistic framing.

Here is what is also true. The scale is one of the least useful measures of progress for an older adult doing Tai Chi. As the forms build muscle through sustained low-load engagement, body composition changes. More muscle, less fat. But muscle is denser than fat, which means the scale may move little, or not at all, while the body is actually getting leaner. A person who loses two pounds of fat and gains two pounds of muscle weighs exactly the same on a scale but has a fundamentally different body. The number lies. Clothing fit, energy, balance, and the ease of getting up from a chair do not.

This is not an excuse for the scale not moving. It is a description of what is actually happening. The most useful approach is to track the things the scale cannot see. How long can you hold a single-leg balance? How does the walk up the stairs feel on Day 28 compared to Day 1? How quickly does the morning stiffness resolve? These questions answer accurately. The scale answers something different and, at this stage of life, something less important.

What Tai Chi actually delivers over time is a set of changes that precede visible fat loss and are more durable than it. Inflammation decreases. Sleep improves. Cortisol comes down. Muscle is preserved or slowly rebuilt. Insulin sensitivity improves. Each of these changes shifts the body toward a state where fat loss becomes more possible. The practice creates the conditions. The conditions produce the result.

Most people who practice Tai Chi consistently for 28 days and beyond notice changes in energy, sleep, and ease of movement before they notice changes on the scale. Some notice the scale eventually. Some do not notice it much at all and realize at some point that their clothes fit differently. Both are real progress. Neither requires the scale to confirm it.

There is also a psychological dimension worth naming. People who have tried and failed at traditional weight loss approaches, and there are many of them, often arrive at a new practice carrying a weight of self-criticism that has nothing to do with the practice itself. It colors how they interpret early results. It makes them impatient with progress that is real but quiet. One of the things this practice gives back, often before any physical change is visible, is a different relationship with effort. Tai Chi is not punishing. It does not reward suffering. It rewards showing up consistently and paying attention. That shift in orientation, from performance to presence, turns out to matter more than most people expect.

This is a 10-minute-a-day program for a reason. Not because 10 minutes is the most anyone could handle, but because 10 minutes done every day produces better results than an hour done twice a week. Consistency is the variable that matters most. A short practice you actually complete beats an ambitious one you skip. Start with 10 minutes. Stay with it. The practice grows at its own pace.

Chapter 2

How Tai Chi Burns Fat

People ask this question with a skeptical look. You are moving slowly. You are not out of breath. You are not sweating through your shirt. How is this burning fat?

It is a fair question, and the answer requires a small adjustment in how you think about the relationship between exercise and fat loss.

The Metabolism Connection

Resting metabolic rate is the number of calories your body burns doing nothing. Just keeping organs running, maintaining temperature, breathing. This accounts for roughly sixty to seventy percent of your total daily calorie burn, far more than any exercise session. The most powerful thing you can do to support fat loss is to protect and build your resting metabolic rate.

Muscle is metabolically expensive tissue. It burns calories at rest in a way that fat tissue does not. Every pound of muscle you maintain or add burns additional calories every single day without you doing anything specific. Tai Chi preserves and slowly rebuilds muscle mass in the legs, core, and upper body through sustained low-load engagement. This is not the dramatic muscle gain of weightlifting. It is the kind of steady functional muscle that keeps the metabolism running at a higher rate and makes everyday physical tasks easier.

For people over sixty who have lost muscle gradually over the previous decade without fully noticing, this rebuilding process produces compounding returns. More muscle means a higher resting metabolic rate, which means more calories burned at rest, which means the same food intake produces less fat accumulation. The body's composition shifts even when the weight on the scale does not, because the ratio of metabolically active tissue to stored fat is changing. This is the mechanism behind the familiar observation that long-term Tai Chi practitioners tend to look leaner and move more easily than their age and scale weight would predict.

Non-exercise activity thermogenesis, sometimes called NEAT, is the energy your body uses for all the physical activity that is not formal exercise: walking to the kitchen, shifting position in a chair, carrying groceries. People with better muscle tone and better energy levels move more throughout the day, not just during workouts, and this accumulated movement accounts for a significant portion of daily calorie burn. Tai Chi practitioners consistently report higher energy levels and more ease of movement, which translates directly to more NEAT and a higher total daily energy expenditure.

The practical implication is that the benefit of a 10-minute Tai Chi session extends well beyond those 10 minutes. The improved energy and reduced fatigue that follow practice produce more spontaneous movement throughout the rest of the day. More standing, more walking, more willingness to take the stairs. None of these individual choices is dramatic. Together they represent a meaningful shift in total daily energy expenditure that compounds over weeks and months into something the scale eventually notices. This is one of the reasons practitioners consistently report feeling more active generally, not just during the formal practice period.

Additionally, slow sustained movement like Tai Chi relies on fat oxidation as a primary fuel source. The body uses fat stores preferentially for lower-intensity sustained activity. Short intense bursts rely more on glucose. If fat metabolism is the goal, the pace of Tai Chi is not a disadvantage. It is a feature. This is one of the reasons the practice produces fat loss effects in people who have not responded to higher-intensity approaches: it targets the fat-burning pathway directly, without the cortisol cost of more aggressive exercise.

There is a useful way to think about this distinction. Intense exercise is a withdrawal from the body's energy account. The body responds by defending that account more aggressively, storing more conservatively, and demanding more rest to recover. Moderate sustained exercise is more like gentle interest drawn on the same account. The body does not defend against it. It adapts to it. Over weeks and months, the adaptation produces a body that is better at accessing its fat stores, more efficient at recovery, and more capable of sustaining the practice that produces those adaptations. That compounding process is what the 28-day program initiates.

Cortisol, Stress, and Stubborn Fat

This is the connection that most exercise books skip over, and it explains something that frustrates many people over sixty: they eat carefully, they exercise when they can, and the fat around their midsection stays exactly where it is.

Cortisol is the body's primary stress hormone. In appropriate amounts it is useful: it mobilizes energy, sharpens focus, and prepares the body for action. The problem is chronic elevation. When cortisol stays elevated over weeks and months, from persistent stress, poor sleep, overtraining, or underlying anxiety, it drives a specific pattern of fat storage. Abdominal fat. Visceral fat. The kind that sits in and around the organs and is most associated with metabolic disease.

Chronically elevated cortisol also suppresses testosterone and growth hormone, both of which are already declining with age. It disrupts insulin signaling, making the body less efficient at using glucose for energy and more likely to store it as fat. And it elevates inflammatory markers throughout the body, creating a low-grade systemic inflammation that further slows metabolism and impairs recovery.

Multiple published clinical studies have shown that regular Tai Chi practice measurably lowers cortisol levels. The mechanism involves both the slow rhythmic movement itself and the diaphragmatic breathing that runs through every session. Deep abdominal breathing activates the vagus nerve, which stimulates the parasympathetic nervous system. When the parasympathetic system is active, cortisol production decreases. Heart rate drops. Blood pressure drops. The body moves out of the stress state it may have been living in for years.

For a person whose stubborn abdominal fat is being driven by chronically elevated cortisol, ten minutes of Tai Chi practice is not just exercise. It is a direct physiological intervention on the mechanism causing the problem. This is what other exercise forms often miss, and why some people who try harder with conventional exercise see diminishing returns while Tai Chi practitioners report visible changes in body composition without extreme effort.

The cortisol reduction is not subtle or slow. Studies measuring salivary cortisol before and after single Tai Chi sessions have documented reductions within a single practice. The cumulative effect over weeks of daily practice is correspondingly larger. For people who have been living with elevated stress, poor sleep, and the particular kind of tiredness that does not resolve with rest, this shift in the hormonal environment is often the first thing they notice. Not fat loss. Not strength. A quieter nervous system. That quieter state is the foundation everything else builds on.

It is worth being direct about what this means practically. Addressing abdominal fat accumulation by lowering cortisol through daily practice is not the same as burning calories during a workout. It is intervening at the hormonal level that decides where fat is stored in the first place. This is why the approach works when higher-intensity exercise does not, and why the people who struggle most with stubborn belly fat despite doing everything else right are often the same people who respond most clearly to Tai Chi.

Muscle, Movement, and the 10-Minute Window

There is good evidence that the timing and consistency of movement matters as much as the volume. A daily 10-minute practice produces different physiological effects than a single one-hour session per week, even if the total time is similar.

One reason is insulin sensitivity. After a session of moderate sustained movement, the muscles become more receptive to glucose uptake for several hours. The glucose that enters the blood after a meal gets routed into muscle cells rather than converted to fat. This effect is real but time-limited. It peaks in the hours following practice and fades. Daily practice keeps this window open consistently, while infrequent practice does not.

Another reason is the cortisol regulation effect. A single session lowers cortisol for hours. Daily sessions begin to shift the baseline. Over weeks of consistent practice, the resting cortisol level itself tends to decrease. This is a cumulative effect that requires regularity, not intensity. The body responds to the pattern more than to the volume.

The muscle activation pattern in Tai Chi also deserves specific attention. The soft-bend position held throughout the forms, knees slightly bent, weight partially supported by the leg muscles for the entire session, is a form of sustained isometric and isotonic work that is particularly effective for the quadriceps, gluteal muscles, and core stabilizers. These are precisely the muscle groups most responsible for resting metabolic rate, functional strength, and fall prevention. A 10-minute session of Tai Chi in this position is not a casual stroll. It is sustained targeted muscle engagement for the full duration.

For older adults specifically, the recovery profile of short consistent sessions is far more manageable than infrequent longer ones. The body does not need to recover from 10 minutes of Tai Chi the way it needs to recover from an hour-long cardio class. You can show up every day without accumulating the kind of physical debt that leads to skipped sessions. The program is built around this principle. Ten minutes a day, every day, produces better compounding results over 28 days than any less frequent approach at the same total weekly volume.

What "Feeling Younger" Looks Like in the Body

The phrase 'feel younger' gets used often in the marketing around senior fitness, usually vaguely enough that it means nothing in particular. Here is what it actually refers to when it is real.

Proprioception improves.

Proprioception is the body's internal sense of its own position in space. It is what tells you where your foot is without looking at it, what maintains your balance when the ground shifts, what prevents a stumble on an uneven sidewalk from becoming a fall. Proprioception declines with age and is significantly improved by Tai Chi practice, which constantly challenges balance and weight distribution in controlled safe ways. Better proprioception means you move through the world with more confidence and less caution.

The improvement in proprioception shows up first in small daily moments. Reaching across a counter and not needing to steady yourself. Turning around quickly without pausing. Managing a step down in dim light without bracing. These are not dramatic events, but their accumulation changes the experience of being in a body that is aging. The practice gives them back one small moment at a time.

Joint inflammation decreases.

The slow sustained movement of Tai Chi stimulates synovial fluid production in the joints. This fluid reduces friction and inflammation. Many people in their first two weeks of practice notice that the stiffness they carry in the morning begins to resolve more quickly. Within a month, some notice it has reduced significantly. The joints feel more like they used to. That is the synovial fluid doing its job.

Sleep quality improves.

The cortisol reduction effect and the physical fatigue of consistent movement both contribute to better sleep. Better sleep in turn lowers cortisol, supports growth hormone production, and allows the body to perform the cellular repair that happens during deep sleep. Sleep and movement reinforce each other in a cycle that, once established, becomes self-sustaining. For people who have struggled with disrupted sleep for years, the improvement is often one of the first and most welcome changes they notice.

Circulation improves.

The sustained whole-body movement of Tai Chi increases blood flow throughout the body, including to the extremities and the brain. Many practitioners report a sense of mental clarity following practice that they do not experience after other types of exercise. This is partly the mental focus effect of the practice itself, and partly improved cerebral circulation. It is not incidental. It is consistent enough that it is worth expecting.

These changes arrive before the scale moves. They are the first signs that something real is happening in the body. When you notice them, and most people do within the first two to three weeks, that is the evidence that the practice is working. Trust it. The scale will do what it does in its own time, and you will be better positioned to understand what the number means when you have already seen what the practice has done to the way you move, sleep, and feel.

Chapter 3

Getting Ready

Before the first movement, before the first session, there are a few things worth getting right. They don't take long. But the people who do them tend to stay with this program. The ones who skip them often don't.

Your Space, Your Chair, Your Shoes

The people I've watched struggle most in the first week of a new movement practice are almost never struggling with the movements. They're struggling with the setup. They do the first session in a cramped hallway with a rolling chair and thick socks on a slippery floor, and then wonder why nothing felt right. So let's handle this now, once, and not have to think about it again.

Your Space

You need a rectangular floor area roughly six feet long and four feet wide. That's it. Push back the coffee table, move a dining chair to the side, clear a corner of the bedroom. The space doesn't need to be special. It needs to be clear. You should be able to extend both arms fully to each side without touching anything, and step forward and back four or five times without hitting furniture.

If you can see outside from your practice space, that's a small advantage. Natural light and something to look at in the middle distance helps with balance work. But a plain wall will do the same job. The only thing that matters is that the floor is non-slip, flat, and free.

Your Chair

The chair is for the seated modifications in every exercise. It is not optional. Every standing movement in this book has a seated version, and you'll want access to the chair even on days when you plan to do everything standing, because some days your body will make a different decision mid-session.

The chair you want is a standard dining or kitchen chair: armless, firm seat, four legs that don't wobble. The back of the chair is for visual reference and occasional steadying, not for leaning. You'll sit toward the front of the seat in the modifications, so a deep armchair or a recliner doesn't work well. A barstool is too high. A folding chair on a smooth floor can slide.

Position the chair at the edge of your practice space, within one step. You don't need to be near it for the standing practice, but you want to be able to reach it without hunting for it.

Your Shoes

Flat shoes or bare feet. That is the full list. Running shoes with thick cushioned soles reduce the feedback from the floor that Tai Chi depends on. When you can feel the floor through your feet, your body makes automatic adjustments in balance and weight distribution. When the sole between you and the floor is two inches of foam, those adjustments are harder to make.

Thin canvas shoes, flat slippers, yoga socks with grip on the sole, or bare feet on a non-slip surface all work well. If you have conditions that require specific footwear, wear what your doctor or podiatrist has prescribed. Don't experiment with that.

That's the setup. If you have all three, you have everything this program needs.

Posture and Breathing

Tai Chi has a lot of movements. But underneath all of them, there are really only two fundamental skills: standing in a useful way and breathing in a useful way. Every form in Chapter 4 is built on these two things. If you spend time with them now, before the program begins, the movements will make sense in a way they can't if you go straight to the forms.

The Tai Chi Neutral Stance

This is what standing well looks like in this practice. It's not military posture. It's not slouched. It is a specific, relaxed alignment that your body can hold for ten minutes without fighting itself.

Feet are shoulder-width apart. Toes angle outward slightly, no more than 15 degrees. Knees are soft, never locked. Your tailbone drops very slightly downward rather than tucking under hard or sticking out behind you. The result is a gentle natural curve in the lower back, not an exaggerated arch and not a flat plank. The spine lengthens upward from that base. Shoulders drop and move back just slightly, away from the ears. The chin is level with the floor. The gaze is forward and soft, at eye height.

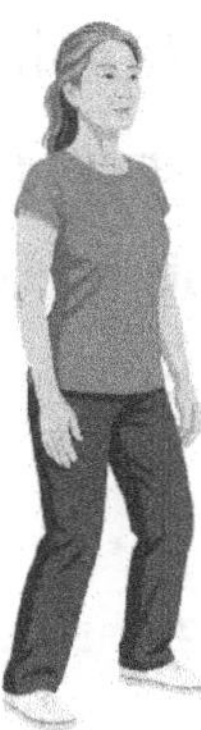

Most people find one or two elements that need attention. Locked knees are the most common. Raised shoulders are close behind. When you first stand this way, it may feel slightly unfamiliar. That unfamiliarity is normal and it fades within a few sessions.

Foundational Breathing Practice

This is the breath that runs through every Tai Chi session. Learning it now means it will be available to you automatically once the movement begins.

Starting Position:

Stand in the Tai Chi neutral stance described above. Rest one hand flat on your lower abdomen, just below the navel, with your other hand on top. This hand position tells you immediately whether the breath is reaching the belly or staying in the chest.

Steps:

1. Exhale first. Let the air leave your lungs completely through slightly parted lips. Allow the belly to draw gently inward as the air goes out.

2. Begin the inhale through the nose. Let it be slow and deliberate. Breathe into your belly first feel your hands push outward as the abdomen expands. The chest should rise only slightly after the belly moves.

3. Continue the inhale for a slow count of four. Belly expands, lower ribs widen, chest rises last.

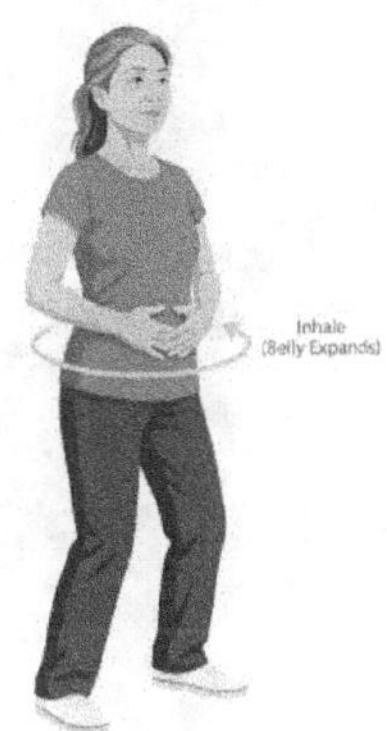

4. Pause for one count at the top of the breath. Don't force the hold. Just a natural pause before the turn.

5. Exhale through slightly parted lips for a slow count of six. Let the belly fall inward. Feel the ribs narrow. Keep the shoulders level throughout.

6. Pause for one count at the bottom before beginning the next inhale.

7. Complete five full breath cycles this way. After the fifth exhale, let the breath return to its natural rhythm without counting.

BREATHING: The breath IS the exercise here. Inhale for four counts. Exhale for six. The longer exhale activates the parasympathetic nervous system this is the mechanism by which Tai Chi practice reduces cortisol.

FEEL IT: After the third or fourth cycle, you will likely notice a slight warmth across the chest and a quieting sensation. Some people feel their hands stop noticeably on the inhale and drop back on the exhale. That is the breath doing what it is supposed to do.

IF NEEDED: If counting feels forced, drop the count and simply breathe slowly. Belly in, belly out. Exhale longer than you inhale. The ratio matters more than the specific numbers.

SEATED MODIFICATION
Sit toward the front half of your chair, feet flat on the floor hip-width apart, spine gently upright without leaning on the chair back. Place your hands on your lower abdomen the same way. The breathing sequence is identical. Many people actually find it easier to feel the belly breath when seated, because the hips and lower back are supported.

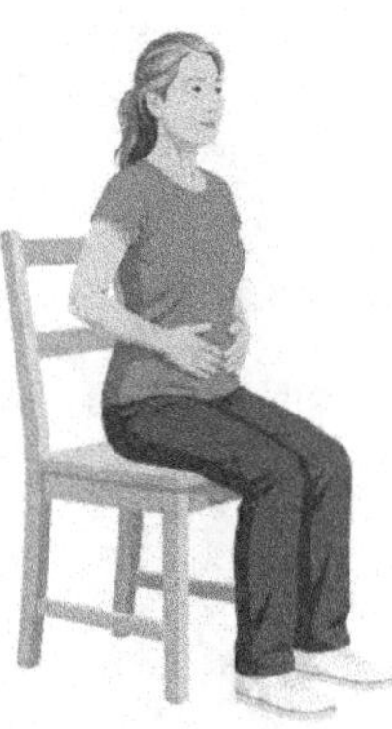

Jing's Note: *You can do this breathing practice any time, anywhere. Two minutes before a difficult conversation. Lying in bed before sleep. In the car before going into a situation you're not looking forward to. The breath does not stop working just because you're not in a Tai Chi session.*

How to Warm Up Without Wearing Out

Most warm-up routines are designed for people in their thirties. They involve big range-of-motion swings and rapid movements intended to raise the heart rate fast. That kind of warm-up is not what this practice needs, and it is not what your body needs at this stage.

The warm-up sequence below takes five minutes. It begins at the top of the body and works downward, preparing the joints systematically without loading them. You will use this exact sequence before every session in the 28-day program. Learn it now, and by Day 3 you won't need to look at the instructions again.

Warm-Up 1: Neck and Shoulder Release

Releases accumulated tension in the neck and upper shoulder girdle and wakes up the vestibular system before balance work begins.

Starting Position:

Stand in Tai Chi neutral stance with hands hanging at your sides.

Steps:

1. Drop your chin slowly toward your chest. Feel the stretch along the back of the neck. Hold for two counts.

2. Lift your chin back to level. Roll your head gently to the right, bringing your right ear toward your right shoulder. Do not force it. Hold for two counts.

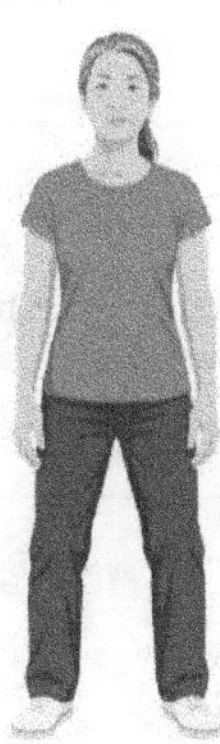

3. Return your chin to the center, level position. Roll to the left in the same way. Hold for two counts.

4. Return to center. Lift both shoulders upward toward your ears on a slow inhale a deliberate, gentle shrug.

5. Roll the shoulders backward and downward in a wide slow circle as you exhale. Complete five circles.

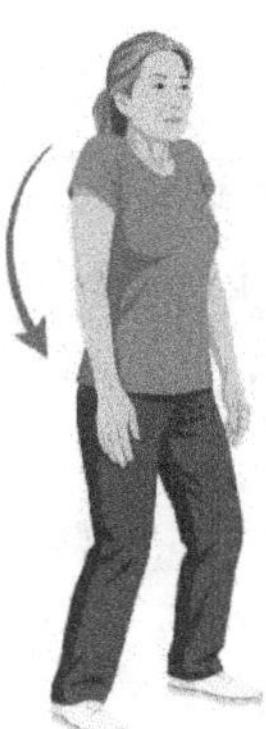

6. Reverse: roll the shoulders forward and upward, then downward. Five circles in this direction.

7. Let the shoulders settle. They should feel slightly lower and more relaxed than when you began.

BREATHING: Inhale as shoulders rise. Exhale as they roll down and back.

IF NEEDED: If neck movement in any direction causes pain rather than gentle stretch, skip that direction. Side tilts and shoulder rolls alone are sufficient.

SEATED MODIFICATION
Perform this entire sequence seated. The neck and shoulder release is equally effective whether standing or sitting.

Warm-Up 2: Wrist and Ankle Circles

Restores circulation and synovial fluid to the wrist and ankle joints the joints most affected by prolonged sitting and morning stiffness.

Starting Position:

Stand in Tai Chi neutral stance. You may rest one hand lightly on the back of your chair for balance during the ankle section if needed.

Steps:

1. Extend both arms forward at hip height, wrists loose, fingers relaxed.

2. Rotate both wrists in slow inward circles, five full rotations.

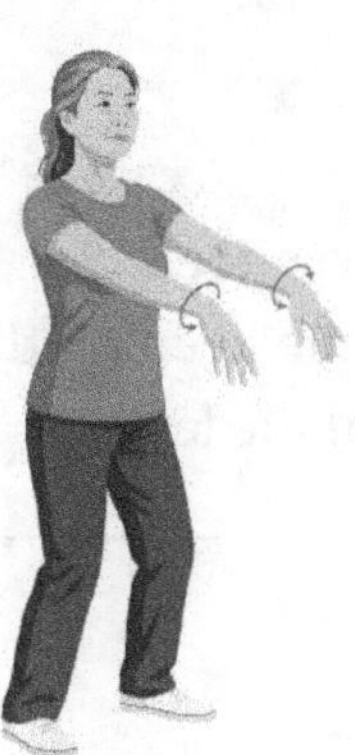

3. Reverse to outward circles, five rotations. Lower your arms.

4. Shift your weight gently onto your left foot and lift your right foot just slightly off the floor heel and toes both up.

5. Rotate the right ankle slowly through its full comfortable range: five circles inward, then five outward. Keep the movement in the ankle, not the whole leg.

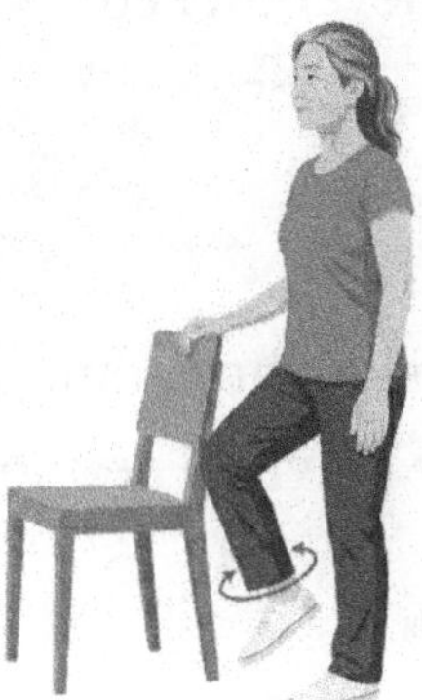

6. Lower the right foot, shift weight, and repeat on the left ankle: five circles each direction.

7. Return to neutral stance with weight evenly distributed.

BREATHING: Breathe naturally throughout. No specific pattern needed for this movement.

FEEL IT: A light warmth in the wrists and ankles after the circles. This is circulation returning to the small joints.

IF NEEDED: If single-leg balance is not yet comfortable, perform the ankle circles while seated. Same benefit, no balance requirement.

> **SEATED MODIFICATION**
> Perform the wrist circles exactly as described. For the ankle circles, keep both feet on the floor and simply lift the right heel while keeping the toe down, rotating through whatever comfortable range you have. Repeat on the left.

Warm-Up 3: Hip Circles

Lubricates the hip joints and sacroiliac area the most commonly stiff structures in people who spend significant time sitting.

Starting Position:

Stand with feet slightly wider than shoulder-width, hands resting lightly on your hips. Knees are soft throughout this entire movement never locked.

Steps:

1. Begin rotating your hips in a wide, slow horizontal circle, as though drawing a circle on the floor with the center of your pelvis. The movement comes from the hips, not the shoulders.

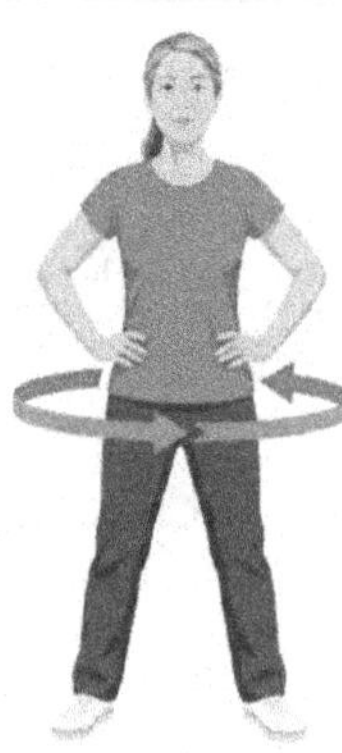

2. Keep the upper body relatively still. Your shoulders and head stay roughly in place as the hips move beneath them.

3. Complete five full circles in one direction. Slow and deliberate, not rushed.

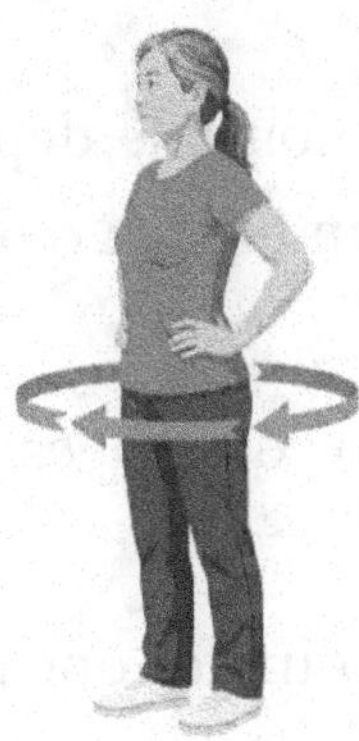

4. Pause for one breath in the center position.

5. Reverse direction for five more circles.

BREATHING: Breathe naturally. If you notice you're holding your breath, exhale completely and let the breath come back on its own.

FEEL IT: A loosening in the hip joints and a warmth along the lower back. People with persistent lower back stiffness often notice it begins to ease after just two or three circles.

IF NEEDED: Reduce the size of the circle if any direction causes discomfort. Even a small rotation produces the synovial fluid benefit.

SEATED MODIFICATION

Seated hip circles work the same way. Sit at the front of your chair, feet flat on the floor, and rotate the pelvis in the same horizontal pattern. The range of movement will be smaller but the joint benefit is equivalent.

Warm-Up 4: Gentle Knee Bends

Activates the quadriceps and gluteal muscles and prepares the knee joints for the sustained soft-bend position used throughout every form.

Starting Position:

Stand in Tai Chi neutral stance with one hand resting lightly on the back of your chair.

Steps:

1. Bend your knees slowly to a comfortable depth no more than a quarter of the way toward a full squat. Most people find 15 to 20 degrees is the right range: thighs slightly engaged, not straining.

2. Keep your heels on the floor. Keep your knees tracking directly over your second toes, not collapsing inward.

3. Pause at the lowest comfortable point for one breath.

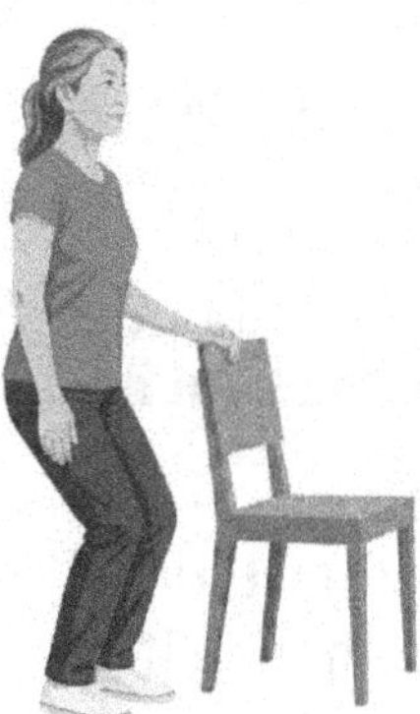

4. Straighten slowly, stopping just before the knees lock at the top. Keep a very slight softness in the joint.

5. Pause at the top for one breath before beginning the next repetition.

6. Complete eight repetitions at a slow, controlled pace.

BREATHING: Inhale as you lower. Exhale as you rise.

FEEL IT: A gentle engagement in the front of the thighs. Not burning working. If you feel sharp pain in the knees at any point, stop and reduce the depth.

IF NEEDED: If knee bends are not comfortable standing, skip this movement entirely during warm-up. The chair sit-to-stand in the Strength Builders provides a safer version when the knees are ready.

SEATED MODIFICATION

Sit toward the front of your chair. Lean slightly forward from the hips, then press through the feet and stand up using the legs without pushing off with your hands. Lower back down slowly and controlled. This is a full version of the movement from a supported position. Repeat eight times.

Jing's Note: *The warm-up takes five minutes when done at practice pace. I know five minutes can feel like a lot before a ten-minute session. But the warm-up is not separate from the practice. It is the beginning of it. The breathing shifts in the first two exercises. The joints open in the third and fourth. By the time you reach the forms, your body is already in a different state than when you started.*

Low-Energy Days, Stiff Mornings, and Bad Knees

Any 28-day program long enough to produce results is also long enough to include days when things don't feel right. The answer is not to skip those days. The answer is to know in advance what you do instead.

Low-Energy Days

On a day when energy is genuinely low, the session changes but does not disappear. Do the Foundational Breathing Practice from this chapter. Do the warm-up sequence, moving slowly through it. Then do Cloud Hands from Chapter 4, just Cloud Hands for the duration of your usual session time. That's it. Three minutes, five minutes, however long it takes. The forms are not what matters on those days. The breath and the movement rhythm are.

Most people find that a low-energy session, done slowly, leaves them feeling better than before they started. Not always. But often enough that it's worth doing every time.

Stiff Mornings

Joint stiffness in the first 30 minutes after waking is normal and has nothing to do with how the rest of your day will feel. Synovial fluid needs movement to redistribute after you've been horizontal for hours. If you practice in the morning, do the warm-up more slowly and with a smaller range of motion than you would later in the day. Don't push into the end of a joint's range when it hasn't had time to open yet. By the time you've completed the warm-up, the stiffness will have largely resolved on its own.

If morning stiffness is severe or takes more than an hour to ease, mention it to your doctor. That's a different conversation than a body that takes ten minutes to loosen up.

Bad Knees

'Bad knees' covers a wide range of things, and they don't all require the same response. If your knees are stiff but not painful during Tai Chi, the practice will likely help them over time. Keep the soft-bend position throughout the forms. Never lock the knees, ever. If the bent position causes pain, reduce the depth of the bend until you find a comfortable range. If any specific movement causes sharp or persistent pain, skip that movement and use the seated version.

What you're aiming for is a position where the knees are working without pain. That position is different for every person. You are the one who knows where that line is.

Your Starting Point Assessment

Before Day 1, take three minutes to do this. It isn't a test. Nothing here has a pass or fail. It's a record of where you are today, so that when you reach the progress checks in Week 2, Week 3, and at the end of Day 28, you have something real to compare against.

Write down your results somewhere. A notebook, the back of this book, a notes app on your phone. The specific numbers are less important than having them to refer back to.

Assessment 1: Single-Leg Balance

Measures current balance baseline. Referenced in the Week 2, Week 3, and Day 28 progress checks.

How to do it:

1. Stand near the back of your chair with one hand available to touch it if needed but not resting on it yet.

2. Shift your weight fully onto your left foot and lift your right foot just a few inches off the floor.

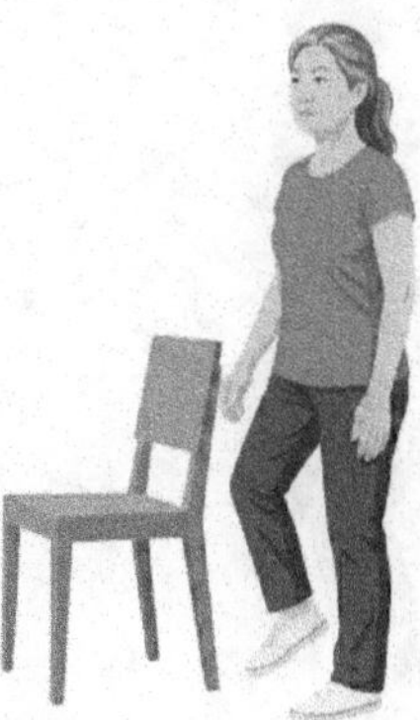

3. Hold the position for as long as you can, up to 30 seconds, without gripping the chair.

4. Note the result: Could you hold it steadily for 30 seconds? Did you wobble but manage? Did you need the chair before 10 seconds?

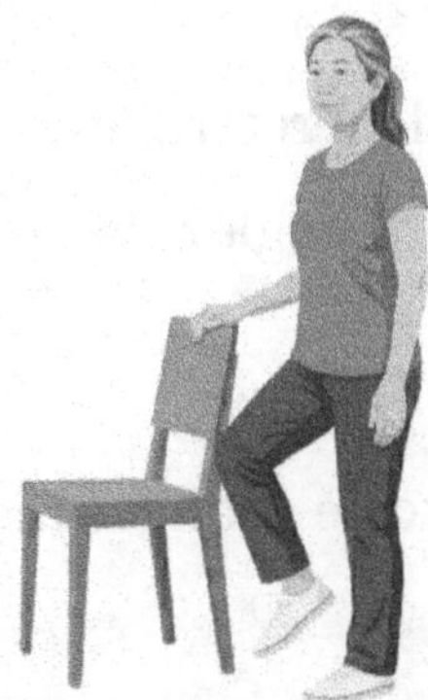

5. Repeat on the right foot. Note the same.

Write down: which side was steadier, and roughly how long you held each side before needing support. That's all.

Assessment 2: Forward Reach

Measures functional flexibility in the posterior chain. Referenced in the Day 28 progress check.

How to do it:

1. Stand with feet shoulder-width apart in Tai Chi neutral stance.

2. Raise both arms straight forward to shoulder height, palms facing each other.

3. Without bending your knees more than they already are, reach forward slowly. Let your body follow your arms into a gentle forward lean from the hips.

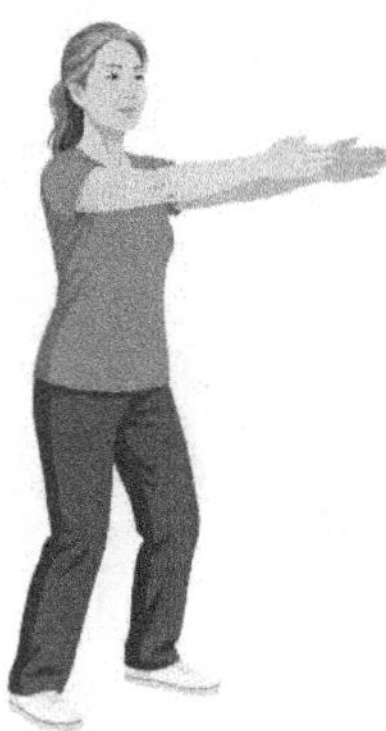

4. Note how far you can reach comfortably before the stretch in the back of your legs or lower back tells you to stop.

5. Hold for two counts. Return to upright.

Write down a simple observation: did you feel restriction early (arms just past level), in the middle range, or only at a significant forward angle? You'll notice if and how this changes.

Assessment 3: Energy Self-Rating

A subjective baseline for tracking the non-scale changes most people notice first.

Answer these three questions and write down your responses:

1. On a scale of 1 to 5, how much energy do you typically have in the first two hours after waking? (1 = very low, 5 = good and steady)

2. On a scale of 1 to 5, how would you rate your general ease of movement over the past week? (1 = stiff and slow most of the time, 5 = moving without much thought)

3. How would you describe your sleep quality this past week, in one sentence?

You will answer these same questions again at the Week 2 progress check, the Week 3 progress check, and at Day 28. The changes in these numbers tend to show up before anything else does.

That's everything you need before Day 1. Your space is ready. Your breathing practice is in place. Your warm-up sequence is learned. You know what to do on the days this is harder. And you have a baseline to measure against.

Chapter 4 is the movement library. Read it before you begin the program. You don't need to memorize the forms you'll have the book in front of you. But reading through them once, following the steps without necessarily doing them, gives your brain a map of where you're going. That map helps on Day 1.

A Small Request

If this book made a difference for you, even in a small way, would you consider leaving an honest review on Amazon or through the website you got a hold of this book?

As an independent author, I don't have the marketing budget of large publishing houses. Reviews are how readers discover books like this. Your feedback truly helps this work reach others who may need it.

It only takes two minutes, and your honest thoughts, positive or critical are genuinely appreciated.

You can leave your review on Amazon by searching the title ***Tai Chi for Weight Loss by Jing Weston*** on Amazon. It takes two minutes, and it matters more than you know.

Chapter 4

The Core Movements

Every movement in this chapter is your program. Learn them here. The 28-day schedule in Chapter Five tells you which ones to do each day you come back to these pages for the full instructions. Read through the whole chapter once before Day 1. You don't need to memorize anything. You just need a first look.

Reading the Instructions

Each movement in this chapter follows the same layout. The starting position is described first in plain prose where your feet go, what your arms are doing, how your weight sits. The image placed after that description shows you exactly what that position looks like. Then the numbered steps begin. Images appear again within the steps at the moment in the movement they correspond to, so you can match what you are reading to what you should be seeing.

Every form ends with three cues: BREATHING tells you when to inhale and exhale through the movement. FEEL IT tells you what correct practice should feel like in the body not what you should achieve, but what the sensation of doing it right tends to be. IF NEEDED gives you a modification if the standard version is too demanding on a given day.

Then comes the SEATED MODIFICATION. It is written in full, with its own image. Not a footnote a complete version of the movement for anyone sitting down. If you practice exclusively from a chair, these seated versions are your forms. They produce the same breathing pattern, the same weight-shift mechanics, and most of the same physiological benefits as the standing versions.

The Strength Builders at the end of the chapter follow the same layout. They are shorter movements, most of them familiar from everyday life, adapted for the specific muscle groups that support Tai Chi practice and fall prevention.

The Seven Foundation Forms

Form 1: Cloud Hands

Trains the continuous weight shift that underlies every Tai Chi movement, warms up the large muscles of the legs, and opens circulation in the arms and shoulders.

Starting Position:

Stand in Tai Chi neutral stance feet shoulder-width apart, knees softly bent, weight evenly distributed. Arms hang at your sides, shoulders relaxed. You will step laterally during this form, so make sure you have two or three feet of clear space to each side.

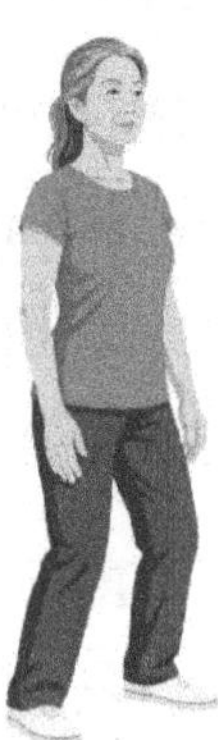

Steps:

1. Raise your right arm in a wide arc up to chest height, palm facing inward toward your body, elbow soft. At the same time, let your left arm rest low at your left side, palm facing gently down at hip height.

2. Begin shifting your weight slowly onto your right foot as the right hand continues its arc to the right, tracing the underside of a wide oval. The left heel may lift slightly as the weight moves right.

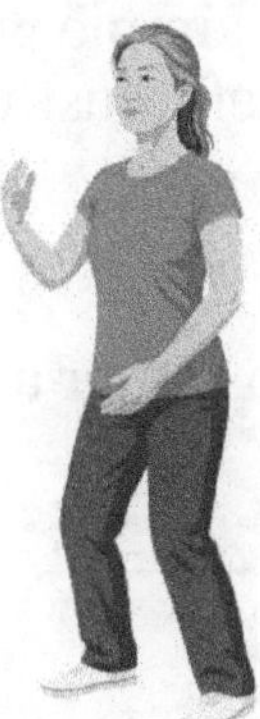

3. As the right hand reaches its furthest point to the right, begin raising the left hand to chest height, palm inward, while the right hand starts to descend.

4. Step your left foot one step to the left as your weight begins transferring onto it. Place the heel down first, then roll onto the full foot.

5. Continue the exchange left hand now at chest height arcing left, right hand descending to hip height. Weight fully onto the left foot.

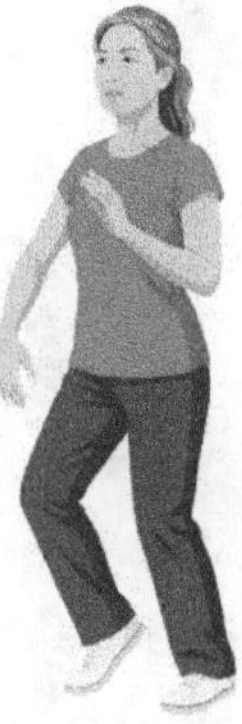

6. Reverse the sequence: step right, shift weight right, right hand rises as left descends. This is one complete cycle.

7. Continue for six to eight full cycles, moving with a slow continuous rhythm. Neither hand stops. The movement flows from one side to the other like water.

BREATHING: Inhale as one hand rises. Exhale as it descends. One full breath per side.

FEEL IT: A continuous warmth developing in the legs from the sustained soft-bend position. The arms float rather than being lifted. The weight shift feels like a gentle tide moving from one foot to the other.

IF NEEDED: Reduce the lateral step to a simple weight shift without moving the feet. Same arm pattern, same breath, same benefit, just without the footwork until your balance is more confident.

Complete six to eight cycles, then return to center and pause for two breaths.

SEATED MODIFICATION

Sit toward the front of your chair, feet flat on the floor hip-width apart, spine upright. Perform the same arm pattern from your seat right arm rises to chest height as weight shifts slightly right in the pelvis, left arm at hip height. Then exchange: left rises, right descends, slight weight shift left. The seated version trains the same arm mechanics and produces the same breath rhythm. The lateral step becomes a gentle pelvic rock from side to side.

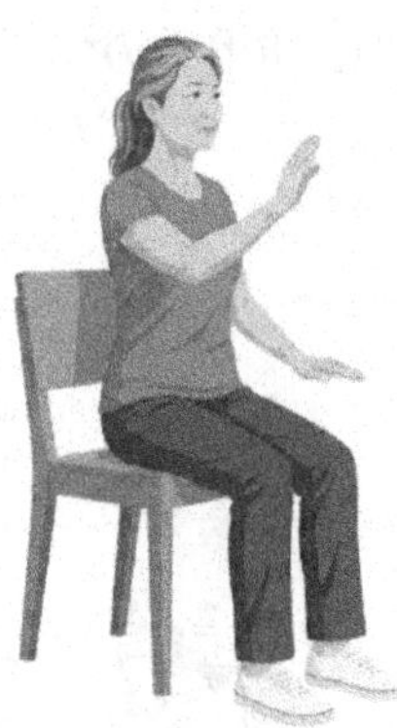

Form 2: Parting the Wild Horse's Mane

A stepping and reaching form that builds leg strength through weight transfer, opens the chest, and trains the coordination of arm and leg movement together.

Starting Position:

Stand in Tai Chi neutral stance with your arms hanging loosely at your sides. You will step forward in this form, so make sure you have four to five feet of clear space ahead of you.

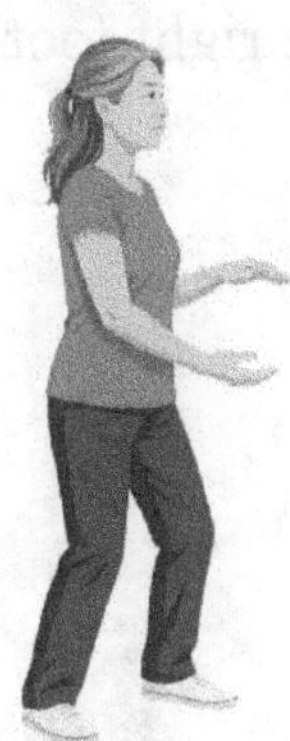

Steps:

1. Bring both hands together in front of your lower abdomen in a 'holding the ball' position right hand palm up below, left hand palm down above, as if cradling a large invisible ball.

2. Shift your weight back slightly onto your right foot, turning your upper body gently to the right.

3. Step your left foot forward and slightly to the left, placing the heel down first at a 45-degree angle outward.

4. As you shift your weight forward onto the left foot, sweep your left arm forward and upward in a wide arc to roughly shoulder height, palm angled upward. At the same time, draw your right arm down and back to your right hip, palm facing down.

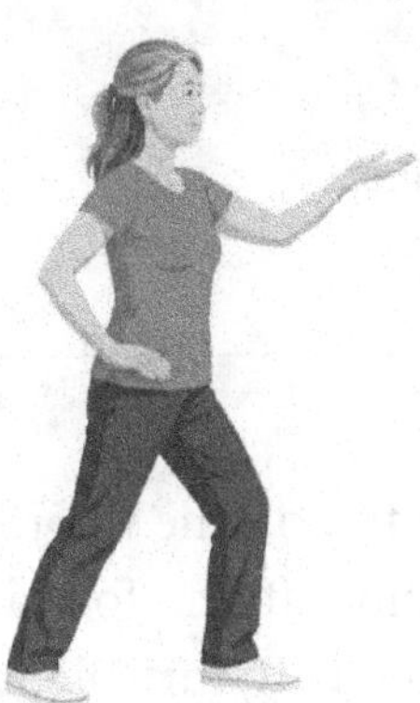

5. Hold the extended position for one full breath left arm forward, right arm back, weight on the front foot, spine upright.

6. Shift your weight back onto the right foot, drawing the left foot back toward center. Regather both hands into the holding-the-ball position, this time with left hand on top for the right-side repetition.

7. Repeat on the right side: step the right foot forward, sweep the right arm forward as the left draws back.

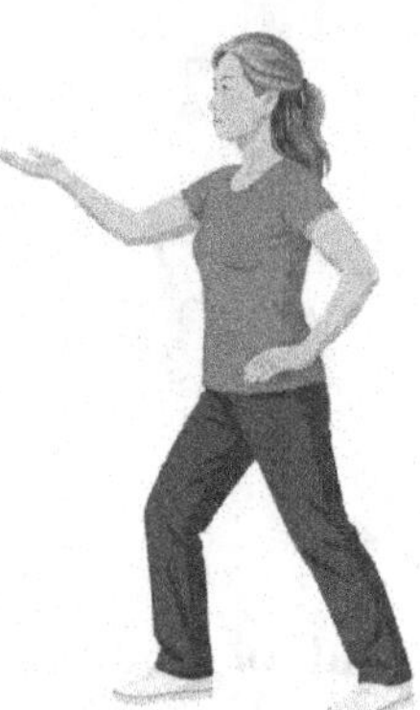

8. Complete four repetitions on each side, alternating left and right.

BREATHING: Inhale as you gather the ball and prepare the step. Exhale as the arm sweeps forward and the weight transfers.

FEEL IT: A lengthening across the front of the chest on the extended side. The back arm creates an opposing pull that opens the chest naturally you don't need to force it.

IF NEEDED: Reduce the step to a half-step if a full step forward is too much for your balance. Keep the arm movement the same.

Complete four repetitions on each side.

SEATED MODIFICATION

Sit at the front of your chair with feet flat on the floor. Bring both hands into the holding-the-ball position. From there, sweep your left arm forward and upward as you draw the right back to your hip, allowing your upper body to turn slightly left. Hold for a breath. Return to center, reverse the ball position, and sweep the right arm forward. This captures the core movement of the form the chest opening and the arm sweep without the footwork.

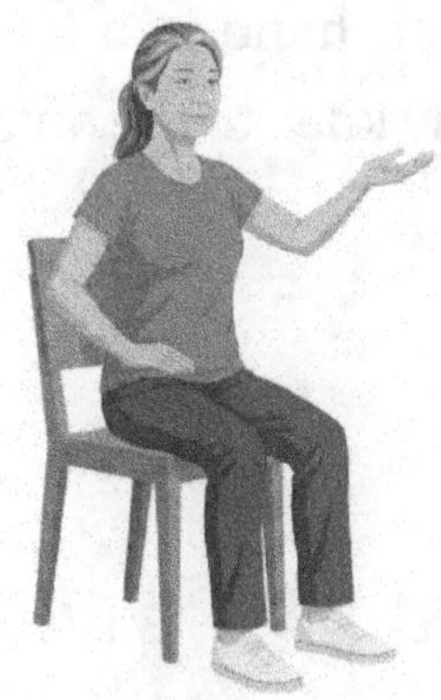

Form 3: Brush Knee and Push

Strengthens the pushing muscles of the arms and shoulders while simultaneously training the hip and waist rotation that gives Tai Chi movements their power.

Starting Position:

Stand in Tai Chi neutral stance. Raise your right hand to the level of your right ear, palm facing forward and slightly outward, fingers relaxed upward. Let your left hand rest at your left hip, palm facing downward.

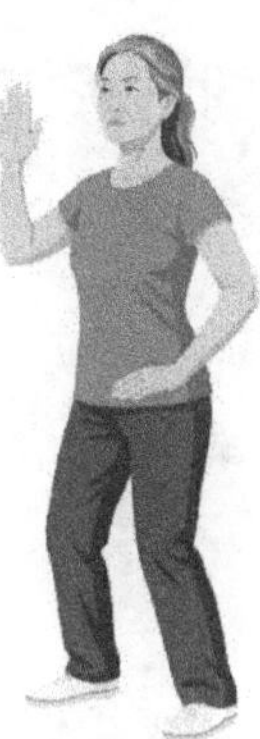

Steps:

1. Step your left foot forward, placing the heel down first. Your weight stays on the right foot during this step.
2. Begin shifting your weight forward onto the left foot as you start moving your right hand forward from beside your ear. It pushes outward, palm leading, fingers pointing up.

3. Simultaneously sweep your left hand in a low arc across the front of your left knee brushing from the inside of the knee to the outside, finishing with the left hand at your left hip, palm down.

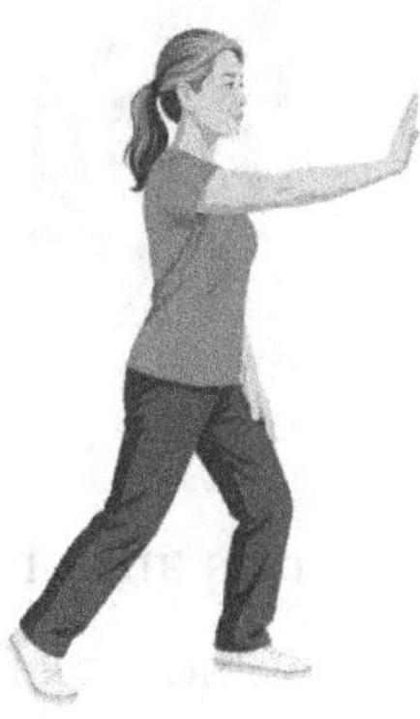

4. Complete the weight transfer so most of your weight is now on the front left foot. The right pushing arm is fully extended but not locked. The left brushing hand rests at the hip.

5. Hold for one breath. Feel the stability of the front leg and the extension of the push.

6. Shift your weight back to the right foot, bring the left foot back toward center, and set up for the right-side repetition: left hand raised beside the left ear, right hand at the right hip.

7. Step the right foot forward and repeat the brush and push on the right side.

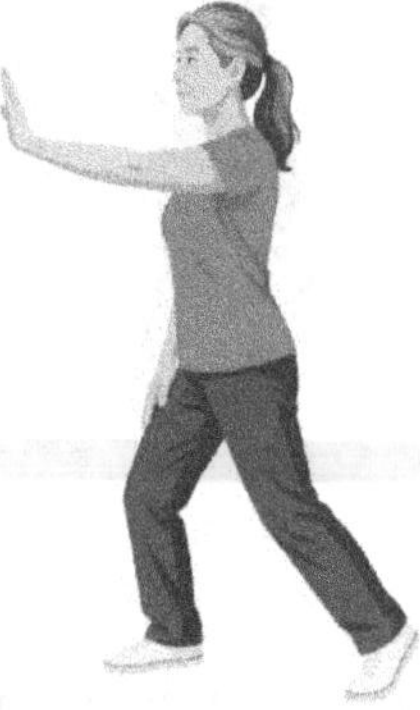

8. Complete four repetitions on each side, alternating.

BREATHING: Inhale as you step and raise the pushing arm. Exhale as the weight transfers forward and the arm pushes out.

FEEL IT: A definite engagement in the front thigh of the stepping leg as it receives your weight. The pushing arm should feel light, not forced the power comes from the hip turn and the weight shift, not from muscular effort in the shoulder.

IF NEEDED: If the step is too demanding, perform the weight shift in place without stepping. The brushing and pushing arm pattern produces the same upper-body benefit.

Complete four repetitions on each side.

SEATED MODIFICATION

Sit at the front of your chair. Raise your right hand beside your right ear, left hand at your left hip. Sweep the left hand across the front of your left knee while simultaneously pushing your right hand forward, palm leading. Return both hands to starting position and repeat on the right side. The seated version practices the arm and waist mechanics without the stepping. Perform four repetitions each side.

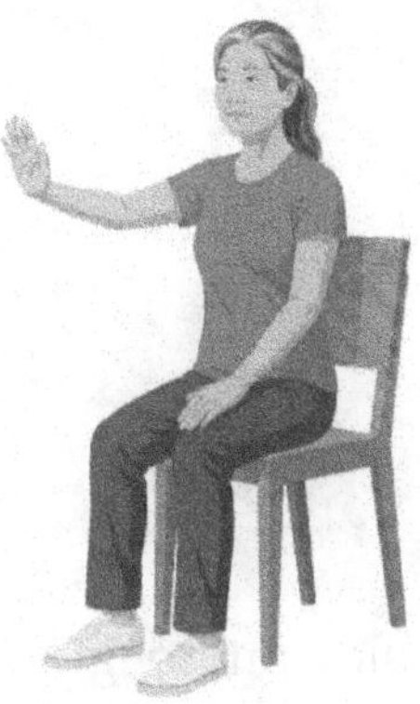

Form 4: Wave Hands Like Clouds

A flowing full-body coordination form that links arm movement, weight shift, and waist rotation into one continuous sequence the closest thing to a Tai Chi meditation.

Starting Position:

Stand with your feet slightly wider than shoulder-width apart. Both hands rest at your waist, palms facing upward, as if you are carrying a tray at hip height.

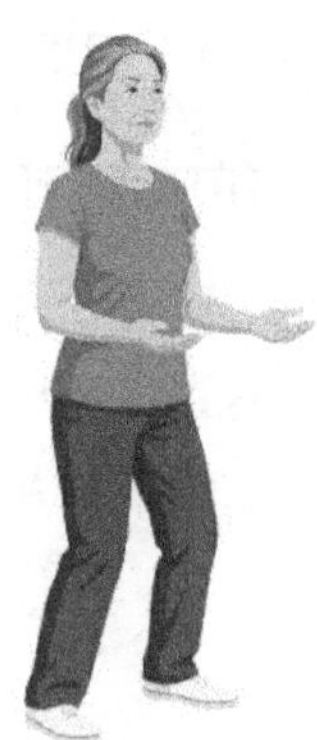

Steps:

1. Lift your right hand slowly in a wide arc out to the right, upward, and then sweeping across the front of the body at chest height, palm facing left.

2. As the right hand sweeps across, let your waist turn gently left to follow it. Your gaze follows the right hand.

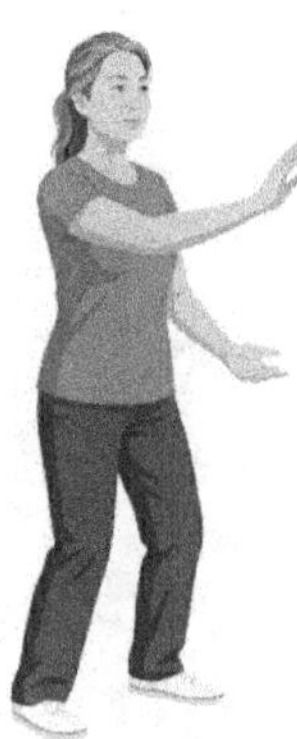

3. As the right hand reaches the left side and begins to descend, your left hand starts its own arc rising from the left hip out and upward, sweeping across the front of the body to the right at chest height.

4. Your waist turns right as the left hand sweeps across. Both arms are now moving in the same continuous oval, one rising as the other descends.

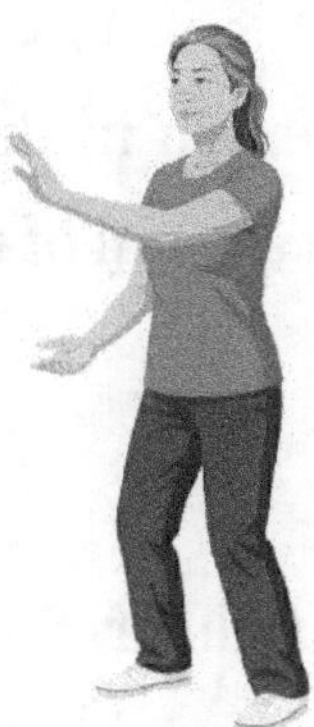

5. Continue this alternating sweep for eight full cycles. Neither hand stops. The waist turns follow each hand as it sweeps.

6. After the final cycle, let both hands settle back to the starting position at your waist, palms up.

BREATHING: Inhale as each hand rises. Exhale as it sweeps across and descends. Your breath will naturally synchronize with the movement after two or three cycles.

FEEL IT: A loosening and warmth through the entire waist and lower back as it rotates. Most people notice this form feels qualitatively different from the others more fluid, less deliberate. That feeling is the goal.

IF NEEDED: Slow the movement down to whatever pace feels sustainable. This form cannot be rushed without losing its effect. Slower is always better here.

Complete eight full cycles.

SEATED MODIFICATION

Sit at the front of your chair with feet flat on the floor. Perform the same sweeping arm movement from your seat, allowing the pelvis to rock slightly left and right as each hand sweeps across. The seated version fully replicates the arm and waist mechanics. If anything, the waist rotation is easier to feel when seated because the legs are not managing balance at the same time.

Form 5: Single Whip

A wide lateral stance form that builds strength in the hips, thighs, and standing leg while training the extended arm position used in several of the more advanced forms.

Starting Position:

Stand in Tai Chi neutral stance. Bring your right arm out to your right side at shoulder height. Gather the fingers and thumb of your right hand together into a loose downward-pointing beak shape fingertips touching, wrist relaxed, the whole hand hanging from the wrist. Your left arm rests at your left side.

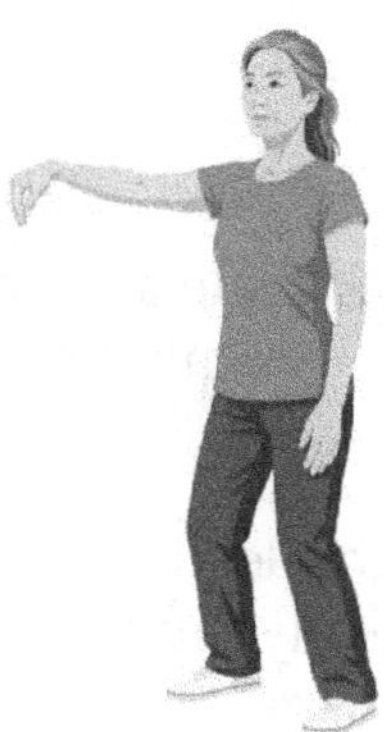

Steps:

1. Simultaneously raise your left arm forward to shoulder height, fingers pointing upward.

2. Step your left foot out to the left wider than shoulder-width bending your left knee as your weight shifts left.

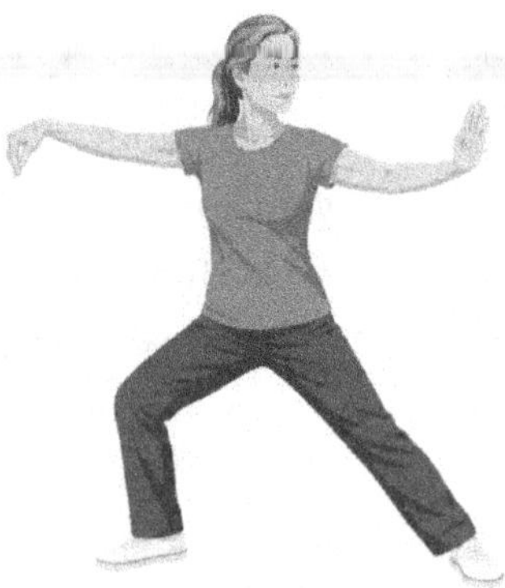

3. Turn your head to look toward your left hand. Your gaze rests on the left palm.

4. Hold this wide extended position for two full breaths. Feel the weight in the left thigh and the opening across the chest.

5. Slowly bring your feet back together, lower both arms, and settle for one breath before repeating on the left side: left arm in the beak position extended left, right arm raised, step right.

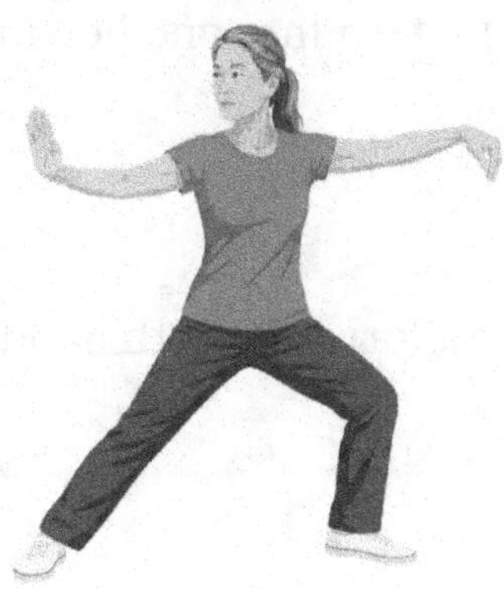

6. Complete three repetitions on each side.

BREATHING: Inhale as you step out and extend. Hold naturally at the top of the breath. Exhale as you return to center.

FEEL IT: A definite engagement in the inner thigh and front of the bent-knee leg. The chest opens between the two extended arms. This is one of the stronger strength demands in the foundational forms it is normal to feel the legs working.

IF NEEDED: Reduce the width of the step so the bend in the knee is shallower. The arm position and the chest opening are the essential elements the depth of the leg bend can be whatever is comfortable.

Complete three repetitions on each side.

SEATED MODIFICATION
Sit at the front of your chair. Extend your right arm to the right at shoulder height in the beak position, fingers gathered downward. Raise your left arm forward at shoulder height, palm facing right. Allow your upper body to turn slightly left as you extend. Hold for two breaths,

Form 6: Grasp the Bird's Tail

A four-part compound movement Ward Off, Rollback, Press, Push that combines every major weight shift and arm coordination pattern into one flowing sequence.

Starting Position:

Stand in Tai Chi neutral stance facing forward. Both hands rest loosely at your sides.

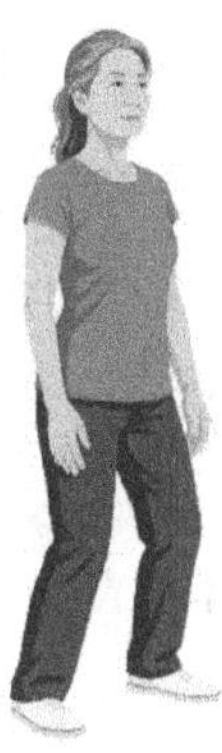

The Four Parts:

Ward Off Part 1:

1. Shift your weight forward onto your left foot as you raise your left forearm horizontally across the front of your body at chest height, palm facing inward. Your right arm rests at your right hip, palm down.

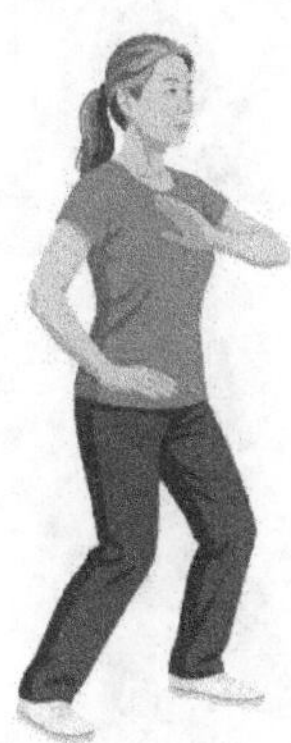

2. Hold Ward Off for one breath. Feel the forearm as a firm but relaxed barrier in front of the chest.

Rollback Part 2:

1. Turn your upper body to the right as you draw both hands back and to the right in a wide horizontal arc, as though pulling something toward you. Weight shifts back toward the right foot.

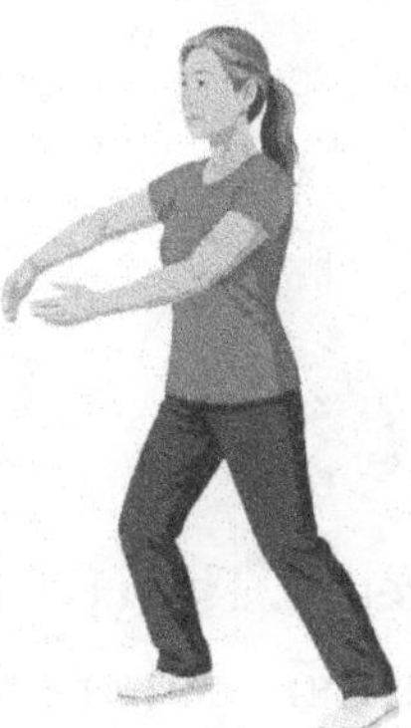

2. Complete the turn so your hands have moved to your right side, weight mostly on the right foot.

Press Part 3:

1. Turn back to face forward. Shift your weight forward onto the left foot. Bring both hands together at chest height right palm pressing against the inside of your left wrist.
2. Press both hands forward together in a smooth arc as the weight fully transfers to the left foot.

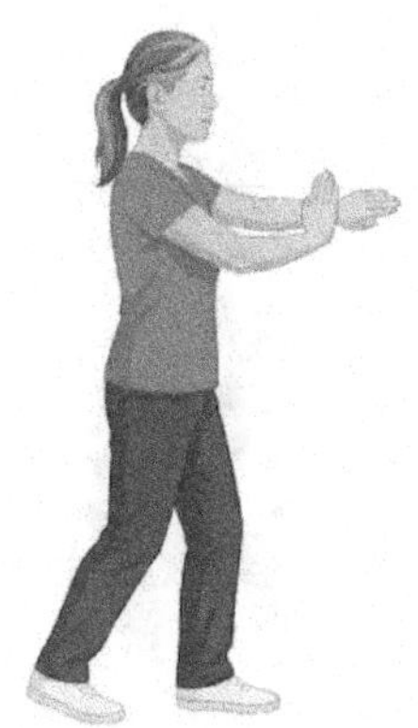

Push Part 4:

1. Separate your hands to shoulder-width. Draw them back slightly toward your chest, then push both palms firmly forward as the weight transfers fully onto the front foot.

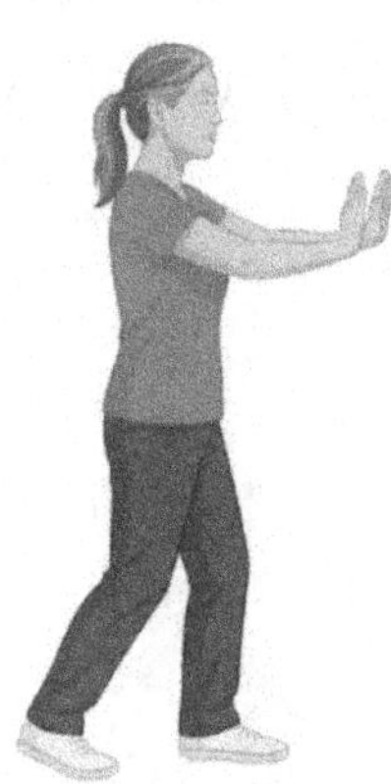

2. Hold the Push position for one breath. Then draw the hands back, shift your weight to the right foot, and prepare for the right-side repetition.

3. Repeat the full four-part sequence stepping onto the right foot. Complete three full sequences on each side.

BREATHING: Each of the four parts has its own breath: inhale on Ward Off, exhale on Rollback, inhale on Press, exhale on Push. This matches the effort pattern of the movement naturally.

FEEL IT: This form is the most complex in the foundational set. In the first sessions, focus on one part at a time. Ward Off and Push alone practiced separately will build the coordination that eventually links all four.

IF NEEDED: Practice Ward Off and Push only for the first week you work with this form. Add Rollback in Week 2. Add Press in Week 3. There is no rush.

Complete three full four-part sequences on each side.

SEATED MODIFICATION
Sit at the front of your chair. Perform each of the four parts from a seated position, focusing on the arm and upper body mechanics. Ward Off: raise your left forearm across your chest. Rollback: turn your upper body right and draw both hands back and right. Press: bring both hands together at chest height and press forward. Push: separate the hands and push both palms forward. The weight shifts become subtle leans of the pelvis. Three sequences each side.

Form 7: Closing Form

Completes every practice session. Signals to the body that the active portion is finished and returns the breath and attention to a settled baseline.

Starting Position:

Stand in Tai Chi neutral stance. This form follows the last movement of your session, whatever it was. Your weight is already settled from the practice.

Steps:

1. Raise both arms slowly forward to shoulder height, palms facing down, as though lifting something light and flat off a table. Inhale through the full rise.

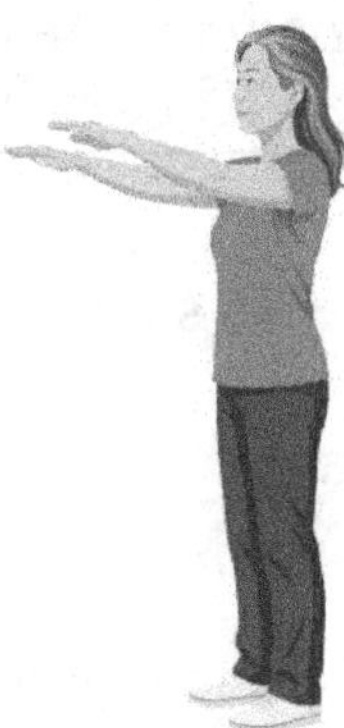

2. Pause at shoulder height for one full breath. Feel the width across the chest and the steadiness in the legs.

3. On the exhale, slowly lower both arms back to your sides, pressing the palms gently downward as though moving through still water.

4. As the arms lower, allow the knees to soften very slightly not a bend, just a release of any residual holding.

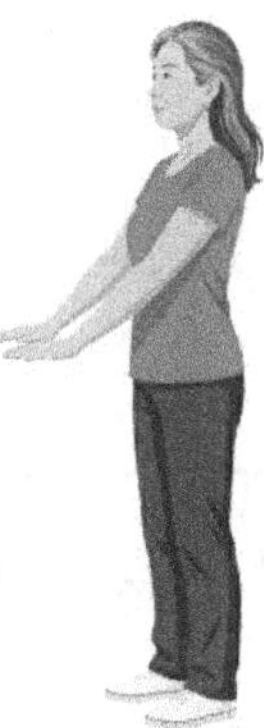

5. Stand still for three complete breaths. Notice what the body feels like after the practice.

6. Let the arms come to rest at your sides. Bring both hands together loosely in front of your lower abdomen right hand over left, palms up. Hold for one breath. Release.

BREATHING: Inhale as the arms rise. Exhale as they lower. Breathe naturally for the three standing breaths that follow.

FEEL IT: A sense of completion the breath returning to its resting rhythm, the body slightly warmer than when you started. Some people notice a subtle lightness in the legs or a quieting of mental noise. Both are normal.

IF NEEDED: If you practice from a seated position, the Closing Form works identically from the chair. Raise both arms, pause, lower them, settle the breath.

Every session ends with the Closing Form. Without exception.

SEATED MODIFICATION

Sit at the front of your chair. Raise both arms to shoulder height as you inhale, then lower them as you exhale in the same slow pressing movement. Sit still for three breaths with hands gathered in your lap, right over left, palms up. Same effect, same intention.

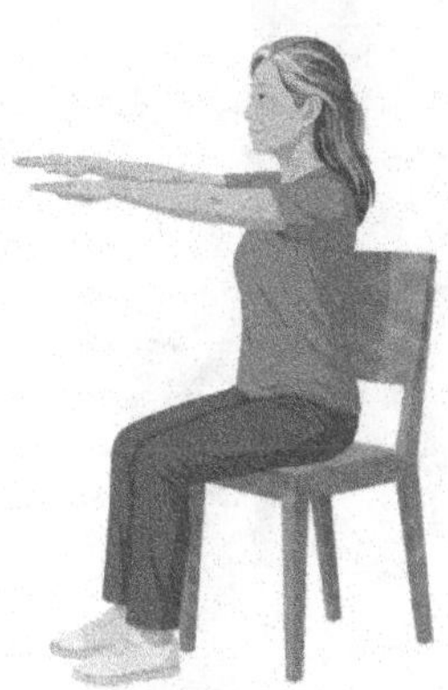

Strength Builders: Where the Muscle Work Happens

These four movements target the specific muscles that support Tai Chi practice and that matter most for independent daily life after sixty: the legs, the core, the upper back, and the postural muscles around the hip. They are not complex. Most of them are simplified versions of everyday movements standing up from a chair, pushing against a wall, rising onto the toes. Done slowly, with control and correct breathing, they build the kind of functional strength that makes everything else easier.

The Strength Builders appear in the 28-day program beginning in Week 3. If they feel like too much in Week 1 or 2, they will not feel like too much by Week 4.

Strength Builder 1: Chair Sit-to-Stand

The single most effective functional strength exercise for the lower body builds the quadriceps, glutes, and core simultaneously using nothing but your own bodyweight and a chair.

Starting Position:

Sit toward the front half of your chair, feet flat on the floor hip-width apart, toes angled slightly outward. Hands rest on your thighs.

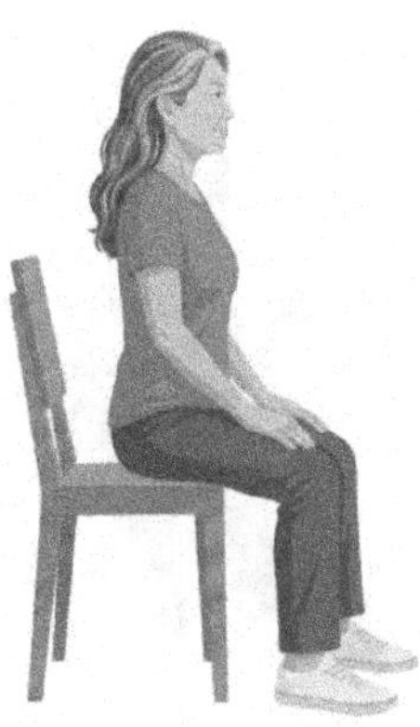

Steps:

1. Lean slightly forward from the hips not the waist so your shoulders come slightly forward over your knees. Keep the spine long, not rounded.

2. Press both feet firmly into the floor and begin standing, using the legs. Do not push off with your hands. Let the leg muscles do the work.

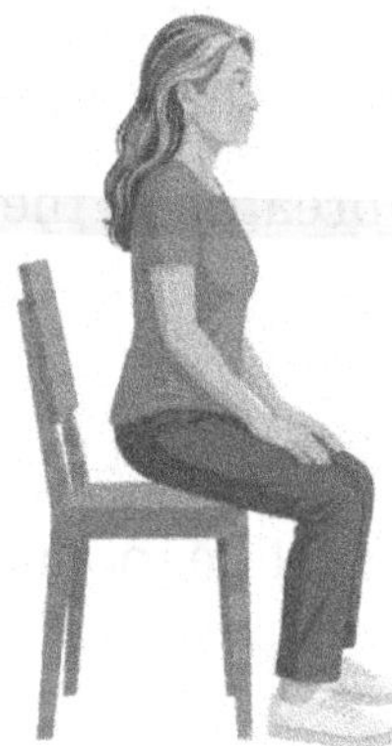

3. Stand fully upright for one breath. Knees soft, not locked. Shoulders back and down.

4. Reverse: hinge gently at the hips, bend the knees, and lower back toward the seat slowly and with control. Don't drop into the chair decelerate.

5. Touch the seat lightly and stand again immediately without using your hands. The touch is a reset, not a rest.

6. Complete eight to 12 repetitions at a slow, controlled pace.

BREATHING: Exhale as you stand. Inhale as you lower. The exhale during the effort is what most people find natural once they try it.

FEEL IT: A clear engagement in the front of the thighs and the glutes on the way up. On the way down, the same muscles work as brakes this is where the strength-building happens.

IF NEEDED: Place your hands lightly on the chair arms or your thighs for support during the first few sessions. Remove the support gradually as the legs grow stronger. If 8 repetitions is too many, start with 4 and add two per week.

Complete eight to 12 repetitions. Rest for 30 seconds and repeat if energy allows.

Strength Builder 2: Wall Push

Builds pushing strength in the chest, shoulders, and triceps using a wall as resistance safer for the wrists and shoulders than floor push-ups, equally effective for this purpose.

Starting Position:

Stand arm's length from a wall roughly two feet away feet shoulder-width apart. Place both palms flat on the wall at shoulder height and shoulder-width apart, fingers pointing upward.

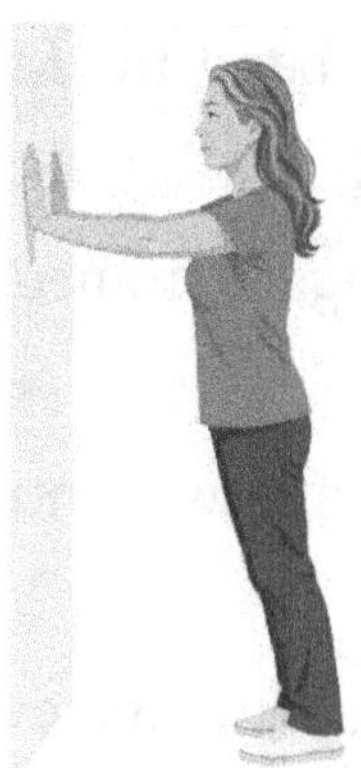

Steps:

1. Keep your body in one straight diagonal line from heels to shoulders no sagging at the hips, no raised backside.

2. Bend both elbows slowly, lowering your chest toward the wall. Keep the body line as you lower.

3. Pause when the elbows reach roughly 90 degrees, or when the chest is two to three inches from the wall.

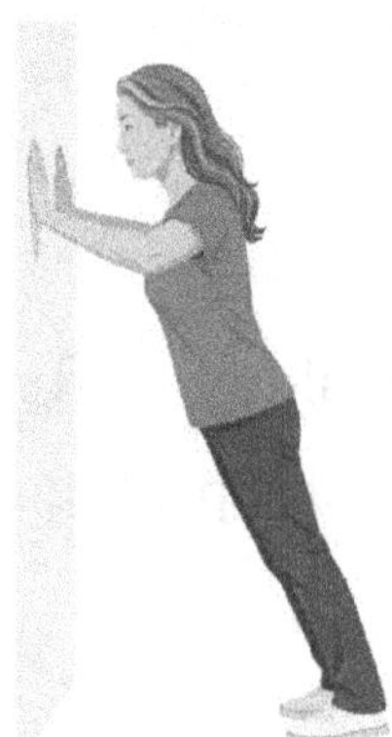

4. Press both palms firmly into the wall and straighten the arms, returning to the starting position.

5. Do not lock the elbows at the top. Keep a very slight softness in the joint at full extension.

6. Complete 10 repetitions at a controlled pace.

BREATHING: Inhale as you lower toward the wall. Exhale as you push away.

FEEL IT: A clear engagement across the chest and the back of the upper arms on the push away. If you feel it in the wrists rather than the upper arms, widen your hand placement slightly.

IF NEEDED: Move your feet closer to the wall to reduce the load. The nearer you stand, the easier the push. Start near and work your way back over several weeks.

Complete 10 repetitions.

Strength Builder 3: Heel Raises

Strengthens the calf muscles and the small stabilizing muscles of the ankle the structures most responsible for preventing falls during unexpected balance challenges.

Starting Position:

Stand behind your chair with both hands resting lightly on the chair back not gripping, just touching for light balance support. Feet hip-width apart, weight evenly distributed.

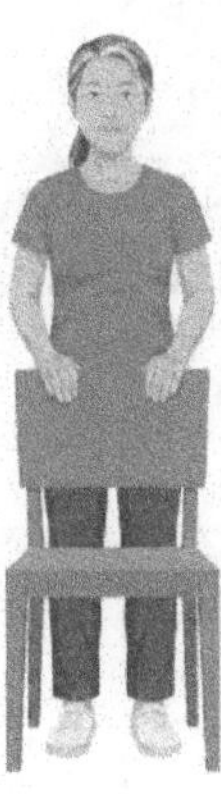

Steps:

1. Rise slowly onto the balls of both feet, lifting the heels as high as is comfortable. Keep the weight even across both feet resist any tendency to roll outward onto the little-toe side.

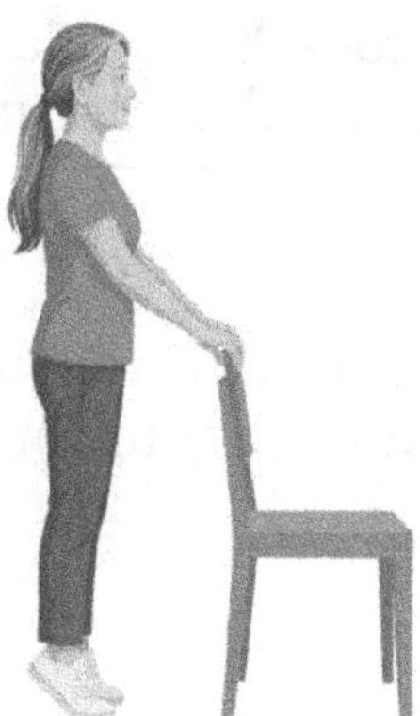

2. Hold at the top for two full seconds. Do not grip the chair it is there for balance only.

3. Lower the heels slowly back to the floor. Control the descent entirely do not drop.

4. Pause with both heels on the floor for one count before beginning the next repetition.

5. Complete 10 to 15 repetitions.

BREATHING: Inhale as you rise. Exhale as you lower.

FEEL IT: A clear burn in the calf muscles after six to eight repetitions. This is exactly right these muscles are typically underdeveloped in people who sit for extended periods, and they respond quickly to this kind of focused work.

IF NEEDED: Reduce the height of the rise if the calves are very weak or if the ankles feel unstable. Even a small raise heels just clearing the floor will build the same strength over time.

Complete 10 to 15 repetitions.

Strength Builder 4: Standing Hip Extension

Targets the gluteal muscles and the lower back extensors the muscles that hold you upright, power your gait, and protect the lumbar spine.

Starting Position:

Stand behind your chair with both hands on the chair back for light support. Feet hip-width apart, weight evenly distributed, knees soft.

Steps:

1. Shift your weight gently onto your left foot without leaning to the left.

2. Slowly extend your right leg straight back behind you, lifting the foot a few inches off the floor. The movement comes from the hip keep the back straight and the hips level. Do not arch the lower back to get more height.

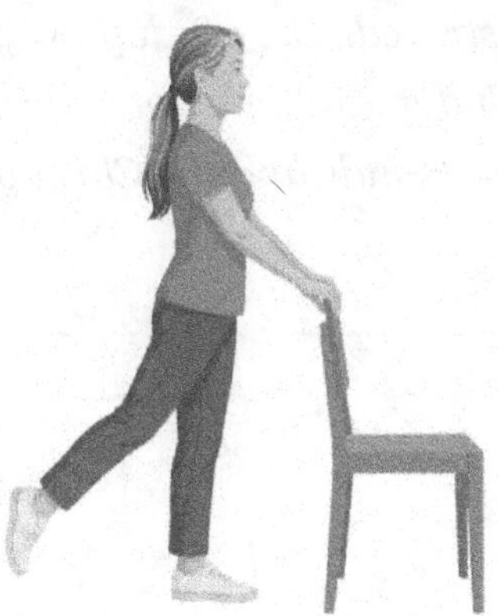

3. Squeeze the right glute at the top of the movement. Hold for two seconds.

4. Lower the right foot back to the floor with control. Do not let it drop.

5. Complete eight repetitions on the right side, then shift weight to the right foot and repeat on the left.

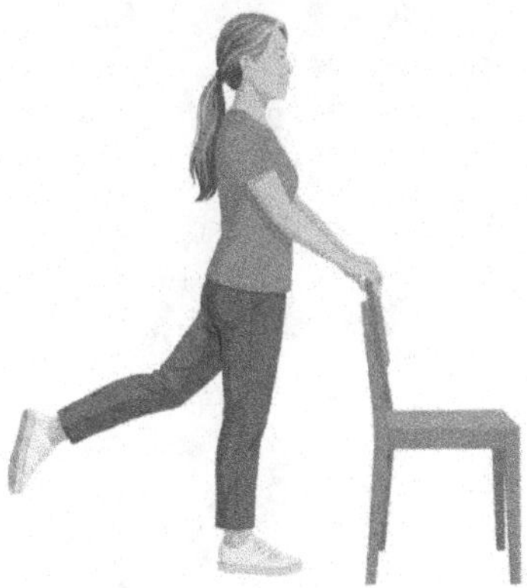

BREATHING: Exhale as you extend the leg back. Inhale as you lower it.

FEEL IT: A distinct engagement in the back of the hip and the upper glute on the working side. If you feel it in the lower back instead, reduce the height of the lift the lower back should not be the primary muscle working here.

IF NEEDED: Reduce the height of the lift to wherever you can maintain level hips and a neutral spine. Even a small range of motion builds the right muscles if the form is correct.

Complete eight repetitions on each side.

> **Jing's Note:** *You now have everything you need to practice. Seven forms, four strength exercises all written out, all illustrated. The 28-day program in the next chapter tells you exactly which of these to do each day and in what order. You don't need to know them all perfectly before you begin. Cloud Hands and the Closing Form are enough for Day 1. The rest will come.*

Chapter 5

The 28-Day Program

This is the working heart of the book. Open it each morning, find the day you are on, and follow the session. Everything you need for each day is on these pages. The movement instructions are in Chapter Four come back here when the program tells you to.

A few things to hold before you begin. Consistency matters more than intensity. A ten-minute session you complete every day produces better results than an ambitious one you abandon by Day 6. If a given day feels too hard, do the low-energy version listed in the glance box. That still counts. It counts fully.

The rest days are not empty. They are in the program deliberately. Each week includes two rest days to support recovery, especially for seniors. The body adapts during rest, not during effort. Skip the rest days and you slow the progress. Honor them and you arrive at the next practice day with more capacity than you had before.

Week 1 – Wake the Body

This week is about beginning, not about performing. You are learning three movements; Cloud Hands, Parting the Wild Horse's Mane, and Brush Knee and Push and the warm-up sequence from Chapter Three. That's all. The sessions are short because they are meant to be completed, not survived.

Most people feel slightly awkward in the first two sessions. That awkwardness is your nervous system registering something new, which means it is paying attention. That is exactly what you want. By Day 5 the movements begin to feel more like something the body already knows, and less like instructions you are following.

+---+
What You Might Feel This Week
• Some joint stiffness in the first session, particularly in the knees and hips. This is normal and resolves within two to three minutes of movement.
• A quiet feeling after the Closing Form that is different from ordinary tiredness. Some people describe it as clearness.
• Mild fatigue in the legs after Days 2 and 3; the sustained soft-bend position is genuinely working the muscles.
+---+

Your Win This Week: Show up every day. The quality of your movement is secondary to the fact that you showed up.

Day 1: First Steps

+---+
SESSION AT A GLANCE
Duration: 10 minutes
Warm-Up Sequence 5 minutes
Cloud Hands 6 cycles
Closing Form
Low energy today: Settling Breath + Closing Form only, 3 minutes
+---+

+---+
Jing's Note: *This is Day 1. You are not expected to do it well. You are expected to do it. Move through the warm-up slowly. Cloud Hands is the only form today. That is all that is asked.*
+---+

+---+
NOTICE TODAY: After the Closing Form, stand still for a moment. What does your body feel like compared to when you started?
+---+

Day 2: Finding the Rhythm

+---+
SESSION AT A GLANCE
Duration: 10 minutes
+---+

Warm-Up Sequence 5 minutes

Cloud Hands 6 cycles

Parting the Wild Horse's Mane 4 reps each side

Closing Form

Low energy today: Settling Breath + Closing Form only, 3 minutes

Jing's Note: *Today adds the second form. Parting the Wild Horse's Mane asks for a step, and that step may feel uncertain at first. Take a smaller step than the instructions suggest if you need to. The arm movement matters more than the step length right now.*

NOTICE TODAY: Did the second form feel harder than Cloud Hands, or about the same?

Day 3: Third Movement

SESSION AT A GLANCE
Duration: 10 minutes

Warm-Up Sequence 5 minutes

Cloud Hands 6 cycles

Parting the Wild Horse's Mane 4 reps each side

Brush Knee and Push 4 reps each side

Closing Form

Low energy today: Settling Breath + Closing Form only, 3 minutes

Jing's Note: *Three forms now. This is the full Week One sequence. The warm-up is five minutes, the forms are five minutes. Ten minutes total. If it runs a little over today while you find the pace, that is fine.*

NOTICE TODAY: Which of the three forms feels least settled? Make a mental note that one gets a little extra attention over the next two sessions.

Day 4: Rest

> **REST DAY**
> No formal practice today. The rest is part of the program.

> **Jing's Note:** *Your body is adjusting to movements it hasn't done before. The muscle soreness you may feel today particularly in the thighs and the outsides of the hips is productive. It means the practice is working. Today the work is rest.*

Day 5: Back to It

> **SESSION AT A GLANCE**
> Duration: 10 minutes
> Warm-Up Sequence 5 minutes
> Cloud Hands 6 cycles
> Parting the Wild Horse's Mane 4 reps each side
> Brush Knee and Push 4 reps each side
> Closing Form
> Low energy today: Settling Breath + Closing Form only, 3 minutes

> **Jing's Note:** *After a rest day, the first movement back often feels more settled than the last session before the rest. This is not imagination. The nervous system consolidates movement patterns during sleep. Trust what you notice.*

> NOTICE TODAY: Does anything feel more natural today than it did on Day 3?

Day 6: Smoother

> **SESSION AT A GLANCE**
> Duration: 10 minutes
> Warm-Up Sequence 5 minutes

Cloud Hands 8 cycles

Parting the Wild Horse's Mane 4 reps each side

Brush Knee and Push 4 reps each side

Closing Form

Low energy today: Settling Breath + Closing Form only, 3 minutes

Jing's Note: *Cloud Hands increases to 8 cycles today two more than last session. Add them at the end. Slow down slightly to stay within the 10-minute window. Slower is always the right adjustment.*

NOTICE TODAY: Feel the difference between 6 and 8 cycles of Cloud Hands. Does the extra time in the movement change anything?

Day 7: Rest

REST DAY
No formal practice today. The rest is part of the program. Use today to recover.

Jing's Note: *Seven days in, the body benefits as much from this pause as from the movement itself. For seniors especially, recovery is part of how balance, coordination, and confidence improve.*

What to Expect This Week

Most people notice two things in Week One that surprise them. The first is that ten minutes is genuinely enough to feel the practice working. Not in a dramatic way in the way that a warm room feels different from a cold one. The second is that the Closing Form, which looks like almost nothing, consistently produces the clearest felt response. The stillness after movement turns out to be one of the most interesting parts of the practice.

What most people do not notice in Week One is fat loss. That is by design. Week One builds the neural pathways that make the movement possible. The metabolic changes come later. Be patient with this week and it will serve the rest of the program well.

Rest and Recovery Getting It Right

Rest days are active recovery, not inactivity. Each week of the 28-day program includes two rest days, especially to support seniors who recover best with regular pauses. Walking is fine. Gentle stretching is fine. What you are avoiding is the kind of effort that would prevent the practice muscles from repairing themselves in time for the next session.

Sleep on rest days matters as much as the rest itself. Growth hormone, which drives muscle repair and fat metabolism, is released primarily during deep sleep. A short night undercuts the adaptation that makes both weekly rest days useful. If your sleep has been poor, treat getting to bed on time as part of the program.

Week 2 – Build the Flow

Week Two adds Wave Hands Like Clouds and Single Whip the fourth and fifth forms. The sessions increase to 12 minutes. The forms you learned in Week One now become the foundation for a longer sequence, and something that was not possible in Week One begins to happen: the movements start connecting. Instead of three separate exercises, you will start to feel a continuous thread running from one form to the next.

This is the week where most people first understand what Tai Chi is trying to do. The flowing quality that distinguishes it from other exercise becomes perceptible once you have enough forms to link together.

What You Might Feel This Week
• The Week One forms will feel more settled almost automatic by mid-week. This is correct. Let them run on their own rhythm.
• Wave Hands Like Clouds may initially feel like too much coordination at once. It isn't. It just takes two or three sessions.
• The 12-minute sessions will feel slightly longer than last week's. By Day 12 they will feel natural.

Your Win This Week: Link all five forms into one continuous sequence without stopping between them.

Day 8: New Form Week

SESSION AT A GLANCE

Duration: 12 minutes

Warm-Up Sequence 5 minutes

Cloud Hands 6 cycles

Parting the Wild Horse's Mane 4 reps each side

Brush Knee and Push 4 reps each side

Wave Hands Like Clouds 6 cycles

Closing Form

Low energy today: Settling Breath + Closing Form only, 3 minutes

Jing's Note: *Week Two begins with a new form. Wave Hands Like Clouds is the most fluid movement in the foundational set it asks for waist rotation in addition to the arm movement. Give it extra time today. The transitions between forms are rough this week, and that is exactly where they should be.*

NOTICE TODAY: Watch what happens in your waist during Wave Hands Like Clouds. Is the rotation happening, or are the arms moving without the body following?

Day 9: Two New Forms

SESSION AT A GLANCE

Duration: 12 minutes

Warm-Up Sequence 5 minutes

Cloud Hands 6 cycles

Parting the Wild Horse's Mane 4 reps each side

Brush Knee and Push 4 reps each side

Wave Hands Like Clouds 6 cycles

Single Whip 3 reps each side

Closing Form

Low energy today: Settling Breath + Closing Form only, 3 minutes

Jing's Note: *The full Week Two sequence today. Single Whip is a stance form it asks for a wider leg position than anything you have done so far. Work with whatever depth of knee bend is comfortable. The arm position and the chest opening are the essential elements.*

NOTICE TODAY: Single Whip is probably the least familiar movement today. Which part of it needs the most attention?

Day 10: Settling In

SESSION AT A GLANCE

Duration: 12 minutes

Warm-Up Sequence 5 minutes

Cloud Hands 6 cycles

Parting the Wild Horse's Mane 4 reps each side

Brush Knee and Push 4 reps each side

Wave Hands Like Clouds 8 cycles

Single Whip 3 reps each side

Closing Form

Low energy today: Settling Breath + Closing Form only, 3 minutes

Jing's Note: *Wave Hands Like Clouds increases to 8 cycles today. This form responds well to volume the more cycles you give it, the more it settles into its rhythm. Slow it down if needed to reach 8 cycles within the session time.*

NOTICE TODAY: Does Wave Hands Like Clouds feel different at cycle 7 compared to cycle 1?

Day: 11 Rest

REST DAY
REST DAY No formal practice today. The rest is part of the program. Use today to recover.

Jing's Note: *Week Two asks the body to coordinate more pieces at once. A rest day here gives the nervous system time to organize the new patterns so tomorrow's practice feels steadier.*

Day: 12 Continuous Flow

SESSION AT A GLANCE
Duration: 12 minutes

Warm-Up Sequence 5 minutes

Full five-form sequence without stopping

Closing Form

Low energy today: Settling Breath + Closing Form only, 3 minutes

Jing's Note: *No form-by-form breakdown today. Warm up, then move through all five forms continuously to the Closing Form. Use the breath as the guide between transitions. If you lose your place, return to Cloud Hands and continue.*

NOTICE TODAY: How far through the sequence did the flow hold before something pulled you out of it?

Day 13: Consolidate

SESSION AT A GLANCE

Duration: 12 minutes

Warm-Up Sequence 5 minutes

Cloud Hands 8 cycles

Parting the Wild Horse's Mane 5 reps each side

Brush Knee and Push 5 reps each side

Wave Hands Like Clouds 8 cycles

Single Whip 4 reps each side

Closing Form

Low energy today: Settling Breath + Closing Form only, 3 minutes

Jing's Note: *Repetition counts increase slightly today. Nothing dramatic one extra rep on three of the five forms. The purpose is to spend a little more time in each movement. Quality over pace.*

NOTICE TODAY: Which form has improved the most since Day 8? It may not be the one you expected.

Day 14: Rest

REST DAY

No formal practice today. The rest is part of the program. Use today's rest to complete the progress check below.

Jing's Note: *Two weeks complete. Today is for recovery and reflection. Use the Progress Check below as part of the rest day, not as extra work.*

PROGRESS CHECK

Take two minutes to answer these questions. Write the answers if you can. Honest answers the program responds to reality, not to optimism.

Can you hold a single-leg balance longer now than on your assessment day? ☐ Yes ☐ About the same ☐ Not sure

Do the Week One forms feel more settled than they did on Day 3? ☐ Yes ☐ Somewhat ☐ Not yet

Have you noticed any change in your morning stiffness over the past two weeks? ☐ Less stiff ☐ Same ☐ Variable

Does the 10-to-12-minute session feel more manageable than it did at the start? ☐ Yes ☐ About the same

Have you skipped any sessions? ☐ None ☐ One ☐ More than one

Week Three introduces the full seven-form sequence and the first Strength Builder. The sessions increase to 15 minutes. If the Week One and Two forms still feel unsettled, continue practicing them at the start of each session before adding the new material.

Increasing Smoothness, Not Speed

The single most common mistake in Week Two is trying to move faster to fit more into the session. Faster Tai Chi is not more Tai Chi it is a different exercise with different effects. The cortisol reduction, the joint lubrication, the parasympathetic activation that makes this practice physiologically distinct all depend on the pace being slow enough for the breath to drive the movement. If you are outrunning your breath, you are moving too fast.

If the sessions are running over 12 minutes, reduce the rep count by one on each form. That is the correct adjustment. Rushing is not.

Week 3 – Burn and Strengthen

Week Three completes the foundational movement set. Grasp the Bird's Tail and the Closing Form join the sequence, bringing the total to all seven forms. The first Strength Builder Chair Sit-to-Stand is added at the end of the practice session. Sessions increase to 15 minutes.

This is the week where the fat-burning mechanism described in Chapter Two shifts into a more consistent state. Three weeks of daily cortisol reduction through diaphragmatic breathing, combined with the muscle activation of the full form sequence, creates compounding effects in the body. Most people begin to feel it in their energy levels around Day 17 or 18.

What You Might Feel This Week

• Grasp the Bird's Tail is the most complex movement in the set. It may take until Day 19 or 20 before all four parts link smoothly. That is a normal timeline.

• The Chair Sit-to-Stand will likely produce noticeable muscle engagement in the front of the thighs. This is productive the legs are doing real work.

• Some people report clearer sleep around Day 16 to 18. This is the cortisol regulation effect building.

Your Win This Week: Complete the full seven-form sequence, including Grasp the Bird's Tail, at least twice.

Day 15: Full Sequence Begins

SESSION AT A GLANCE

Duration: 15 minutes

Warm-Up Sequence 5 minutes

Cloud Hands 6 cycles

Parting the Wild Horse's Mane 4 reps each side

Brush Knee and Push 4 reps each side

Wave Hands Like Clouds 6 cycles

Single Whip 3 reps each side

Grasp the Bird's Tail 2 sequences each side

Closing Form

Low energy today: Settling Breath + Closing Form only, 3 minutes

Jing's Note: *Two new forms today: Grasp the Bird's Tail and the official Closing Form. Grasp the Bird's Tail has four parts Ward Off, Rollback, Press, Push. Practice each part separately before linking them if needed. The session is 15 minutes today. Give the new material the time it needs.*

Day 16: Strength Builder Begins

SESSION AT A GLANCE
Duration: 15 minutes
Warm-Up Sequence 5 minutes
Full seven-form sequence
Chair Sit-to-Stand 8 reps
Closing Form
Low energy today: Settling Breath + Closing Form only, 3 minutes

Jing's Note: *The first Strength Builder joins the program. Chair Sit-to-Stand after the forms, before the Closing Form. Eight repetitions, slow and controlled. The legs will let you know they are working.*

NOTICE TODAY: How does the Sit-to-Stand feel at rep 7 and 8 compared to rep 1 and 2?

Day 17: Full Practice

SESSION AT A GLANCE
Duration: 15 minutes
Warm-Up Sequence 5 minutes
Full seven-form sequence
Chair Sit-to-Stand 10 reps
Closing Form
Low energy today: Settling Breath + Closing Form only, 3 minutes

NOTICE TODAY: Does the practice feel like one thing yet, or still like a sequence of separate pieces?

Day 18: Rest

REST DAY
REST DAY No formal practice today. The rest is part of the program. Use today to recover.

Day 19: Strength Without Strain

SESSION AT A GLANCE
Duration: 15 minutes
Warm-Up Sequence 5 minutes
Full seven-form sequence focus on Grasp the Bird's Tail
Chair Sit-to-Stand 10 reps
Closing Form
Low energy today: Settling Breath + Closing Form only, 3 minutes

NOTICE TODAY: Can you move through all four parts of Grasp the Bird's Tail without a pause today?

Day 20: Continuous

SESSION AT A GLANCE
Duration: 15 minutes
Warm-Up Sequence 5 minutes
Full seven-form sequence, no pauses between forms
Chair Sit-to-Stand 10 reps
Closing Form
Low energy today: Settling Breath + Closing Form only, 3 minutes

Jing's Note: *Same approach as Day 12 in Week Two move through all seven forms as one continuous sequence. The breath connects each transition. If you lose your place, return to the most recent form you remember and continue.*

NOTICE TODAY: How far through the continuous sequence did you get before needing to redirect?

Day 21: Rest

REST DAY
No formal practice today. The rest is part of the program. Use today's rest to complete the progress check below.

Jing's Note: *Three weeks of practice deserve a pause. Rest today, then use the Progress Check below to notice what has changed since the beginning.*

PROGRESS CHECK

Three weeks of practice. Look honestly at each question.

Compare your single-leg balance hold to the Chapter Three assessment. Longer, shorter, or the same? ☐ Longer ☐ Same ☐ Variable day to day

Is morning stiffness resolving more quickly than it was three weeks ago? ☐ Yes, noticeably ☐ Somewhat ☐ Not yet

Has your energy level changed at any point in the day? ☐ More steady ☐ About the same ☐ Too variable to tell

Can you complete the full seven-form sequence without stopping? ☐ Yes ☐ With one or two pauses ☐ Still building

Has your sleep quality changed from your Week One assessment? ☐ Better ☐ Same ☐ Inconsistent

Week Four brings the full practice together all seven forms and two Strength Builders. The sessions increase to 15 to 20 minutes. This is the week where the practice begins to feel like it belongs to you rather than like something you are learning.

Where Fat Burn Shifts Up a Gear

The first two weeks of any new movement practice produce hormonal changes before metabolic ones. The cortisol reduction begins almost immediately measurable changes in resting cortisol are documented within the first two weeks of consistent practice. The fat-burning effects that follow improved insulin sensitivity, increased fat oxidation during low-intensity sustained movement, gradual muscle preservation take longer to establish. Week Three is where the two mechanisms start working together.

This is also the week when the combination of better sleep and lower resting cortisol creates the conditions the body needs to actually use stored fat as fuel. Not dramatically. Not visibly. But consistently, underneath the surface, the metabolic environment is shifting.

Building Real Strength Without the Strain

The Chair Sit-to-Stand is the single most functionally important exercise in the Strength Builder set. The ability to stand up from a chair and lower back down with control uses the exact same muscles as climbing stairs, walking uphill, and recovering from a stumble. Done consistently, it rebuilds leg strength that most people in their sixties have already begun to lose without realizing it.

The goal in Week Three is not maximum repetitions. It is controlled movement through the full range. Eight to ten slow repetitions, lowering all the way to the seat and rising without hand assistance, produces more functional strength gain than 20 half-movement reps done fast.

Week 4 – Feel the Difference

The final week adds a second Strength Builder Heel Raises alongside the Chair Sit-to-Stand. Sessions increase to 15 to 20 minutes depending on pace. Everything else holds: the same seven forms, the same warm-up, the Closing Form at the end.

Week Four is when the practice becomes self-sustaining for most people. The movements are familiar enough that the mental effort of following instructions drops away, and the practice becomes something you actually do rather than something you are trying to do. That shift is the whole point. It is what makes the habit last past Day 28.

What You Might Feel This Week
• The full sequence will likely feel comfortable for the first time not easy, but no longer effortful to organize.
• Heel Raises will produce a clear calf burn. That is the right response.
• Some people feel, around Day 25 or 26, a specific kind of quiet after the Closing Form that is different from any other point in the program. It is hard to describe. You will know it when it arrives.

Your Win This Week: Complete the full practice forms, two Strength Builders, Closing Form on every practice day.

Day 22: Two Strength Builders

SESSION AT A GLANCE
Duration: 15 20 minutes
Warm-Up Sequence 5 minutes
Full seven-form sequence

Chair Sit-to-Stand 10 reps

Heel Raises 10 reps

Closing Form

Low energy today: Settling Breath + Closing Form only, 3 minutes

Jing's Note: *Heel Raises join the sequence today. Ten repetitions, slow rise, slow lower. Place your hands on the chair back for balance not for support. These two Strength Builders together take about three minutes.*

NOTICE TODAY: What do the calves feel like during Heel Raises? That sensation the work of muscles that don't often get directly addressed is exactly what they are supposed to feel.

Day 23: Full Practice

SESSION AT A GLANCE
Duration: 15 20 minutes

Warm-Up Sequence 5 minutes

Full seven-form sequence

Chair Sit-to-Stand 12 reps

Heel Raises 12 reps

Closing Form

Low energy today: Settling Breath + Closing Form only, 3 minutes

Jing's Note: *Both Strength Builders increase by two reps today. This is the target count for the final week. The full session warm-up, seven forms, two Strength Builders, Closing Form is now the complete practice.*

NOTICE TODAY: Does 20 minutes feel different from 10 minutes? What is the difference in how the body feels at the end?

Day 24: Putting It Together

SESSION AT A GLANCE
Duration: 15 20 minutes

Warm-Up Sequence 5 minutes

Full seven-form sequence, continuous if possible

Chair Sit-to-Stand 12 reps

Heel Raises 12 reps

Closing Form

Low energy today: Settling Breath + Closing Form only, 3 minutes

Jing's Note: *Continuous seven-form sequence today the same goal as Days 12 and 20, now with four more sessions of practice behind you. The transitions between forms are the measure. Every smooth transition is a week of work paying off.*

NOTICE TODAY: How does the continuous sequence feel compared to Day 20? Which transitions are cleaner now?

Day 25: Rest

REST DAY
REST DAY No formal practice today. The rest is part of the program. Use today to recover.

Jing's Note: *Near the end of the program, rest is not a setback. It is what helps the final practice days feel more settled, more coordinated, and more sustainable.*

Day 26: Second to Last

SESSION AT A GLANCE
Duration: 15 20 minutes

Warm-Up Sequence 5 minutes

Jing's Note: *Two sessions remaining. The practice is built. What happens on Day 29 is entirely in your hands that question is what Chapter Eight addresses. For now, practice.*

NOTICE TODAY: What part of the practice do you look forward to? Most people find the answer surprising.

Day 27: The Last Full Session

SESSION AT A GLANCE
Duration: 15 20 minutes
Warm-Up Sequence 5 minutes
Full seven-form sequence
Chair Sit-to-Stand 12 reps
Heel Raises 15 reps
Closing Form
Low energy today: Settling Breath + Closing Form only, 3 minutes

Jing's Note: *The last full practice day before the Final Progress Check. Do the session as you have been doing it. No ceremony needed. The ceremony is in having shown up consistently.*

NOTICE TODAY: Is there anything you want to practice particularly well tomorrow on the final day?

Day 28: Rest

REST DAY

No formal practice today. The rest is part of the program. Use today's rest to complete the progress check below.

Jing's Note: *Day 28 is a recovery-and-reflection day. For seniors especially, finishing well matters more than pushing through one more formal session. Use the Final Progress Check to mark what has changed.*

PROGRESS CHECK

The final check. Compare your answers now to your baselines from Chapter Three and from the Week Two and Three checks.

Single-leg balance compare to Chapter Three baseline. ☐ Longer hold ☐ About the same ☐ Varies by side

Forward reach compare to Chapter Three baseline. ☐ Reached further ☐ About the same

Morning stiffness compare to Week One. ☐ Resolves faster ☐ About the same ☐ Improved some days

Energy rating (Ch. 3 Question 1) same scale, honest answer. ☐ Higher than Day 1 ☐ Same ☐ Variable

Ease of movement rating (Ch. 3 Question 2) same scale. ☐ Higher ☐ Same

What happens next is in Chapter Eight. Read it before you decide anything about what to do on Day 29.

Putting the Full Flow Together

By the end of Day 28, most people have a version of the complete practice that is genuinely their own. Not perfect Tai Chi takes years to refine, and the people who practice it for years will tell you it never stops offering new things to notice. But functional. Consistent. Something that has become part of the morning rather than an obligation to manage.

The full sequence warm-up, seven forms, two Strength Builders, Closing Form is a complete practice. It addresses balance, cortisol regulation, muscle preservation, joint lubrication, and cardiovascular conditioning in one 15-to-20-minute session. There is no other widely accessible exercise form that covers that much ground in that amount of time for this population. That is not hyperbole. It is the reason this practice has outlasted every fitness trend of the past century.

What's Actually Changing in Your Body

If you have noticed changes over the past 28 days, they are likely in this order: sleep first, then morning stiffness, then energy, then ease of movement, then balance. Fat loss, if it is happening, is probably last to register consciously and may not yet be visible on a scale even when it is genuinely occurring.

The scale is measuring total mass. Tai Chi practice builds muscle while reducing fat. Muscle is denser than fat. A person who has added a pound of functional muscle and lost a pound of fat weighs exactly the same on a scale while being demonstrably different in every way that matters. Measure the quality of your movement. Measure your balance. Measure how you feel getting out of a chair. Those measures are telling you the truth.

Chapter 6

Eating to Support the Work

This chapter is not a diet plan. There is no calorie count here, no macro ratio, no list of forbidden foods. What is here is a set of principles about food and timing that are specifically relevant to someone doing this kind of practice. They are practical and they are grounded.

No Diet Required What That Actually Means

When this book says 'no diet required,' it means something specific. It does not mean that food is irrelevant or that you can eat anything and have the same results. It means that adding a formal diet on top of a new movement practice is, for most people over sixty, counterproductive.

Calorie restriction as a primary weight loss strategy is already less effective for people over sixty than it was at forty, for the reasons covered in Chapter One: slower metabolism, reduced muscle mass, hormonal changes. When you combine aggressive calorie restriction with a movement practice, the body often responds by protecting its fat stores more aggressively. It reads the combined deficit as a threat and down-regulates the metabolic processes you are trying to support. The result is frustration: less food and more exercise producing less result than either alone, at a cost to energy and mood that makes the practice harder to sustain.

There is also a simpler reason to avoid adding a diet to this program. Starting a new physical practice and overhauling eating habits at the same time is cognitively expensive. Both changes require attention, decision-making, and willpower in the first two to three weeks while new habits are being established. Splitting that energy between two major behavior changes reduces the likelihood of success at either one. The research on habit formation is clear on this: one change at a time succeeds more often than two changes simultaneously.

The practical instruction, then, is this: complete the 28-day program with your eating roughly as it has been. Make the one or two adjustments described in this chapter adequate protein, better hydration around practice, protecting sleep and leave everything else alone until the movement habit is established. Once the practice is part of your daily routine, you will likely find that your relationship with food has already changed in small ways that didn't require effort. That tends to be how the body works when its cortisol is lower and its energy steadier. The appetite signals become more trustworthy. The urgency around food relaxes slightly. These shifts are gradual and real, and they do not require a meal plan to produce.

None of this is permission to eat badly. It is permission to focus on the practice first, trust the process, and let the nutritional adjustments happen incrementally rather than all at once. What follows in this chapter identifies the most important of those adjustments the ones that will directly support what the practice is building and leaves the rest for later, when you have the bandwidth to give them the attention they deserve.

Foods That Work With Tai Chi, Not Against It

The practice asks three things of the body: sustained muscle engagement, efficient cortisol regulation, and consistent energy availability during a short, moderate-intensity session. Each of these has a nutritional corollary.

Protein for muscle preservation.

The most important dietary adjustment for an older adult beginning a movement practice is adequate protein. Muscle tissue is broken down and rebuilt continuously, and the rebuild depends on available amino acids. Most people over sixty consume less protein than their bodies need to maintain muscle mass, and a deficit becomes visible as the gradual loss of strength and body composition that many people attribute simply to aging.

The practical target is roughly half a gram of protein per pound of body weight per day for a 150-pound person, about 75 grams. This is achievable through ordinary food: eggs, fish, chicken, Greek yogurt, legumes, cottage cheese. Not supplements, not protein powder unless preferred. Just consistent protein in each meal. Spreading protein across three meals, rather than concentrating it in one, improves how much the body can actually use. A high-protein dinner with minimal protein at breakfast is less effective than moderate protein at each meal.

For people who are not accustomed to thinking about protein, a practical starting point is simply to make sure every meal includes one of the following: eggs, fish, meat, poultry, legumes, dairy, or tofu. That single habit, applied consistently, will typically move protein intake close to where it needs to be without any counting.

Anti-inflammatory foods.

Tai Chi reduces systemic inflammation through the cortisol-lowering effect of the breath and movement. Certain foods support this process; others work against it. The foods that work with it are the ones most people already know should be on the plate more often: fatty fish (salmon, mackerel, sardines), berries, leafy greens, olive oil, walnuts, turmeric. The foods that work against it are also familiar: high-sugar processed foods, refined carbohydrates, excessive alcohol. No item on that list needs to be permanently removed. The volume and frequency are what matter.

The anti-inflammatory effect of food is cumulative and directional. Adding three servings of vegetables per day and switching from a refined grain to a whole grain produces measurable inflammation reduction over weeks. The goal is not dietary perfection. It is a general trend in a useful direction, maintained consistently over time.

Meal timing around practice.

Practicing on a completely empty stomach is fine for some people and uncomfortable for others. A small snack 30 to 45 minutes before a session something with a little protein and a little carbohydrate prevents the light-headedness that some older adults experience during the sustained stance positions. A hard-boiled egg, a small handful of nuts, a piece of fruit. Nothing heavy. Nothing that competes with the focused breathing the practice requires.

After practice, the window of increased insulin sensitivity described in Chapter Two is real and brief. A small protein-containing snack or meal within 30 to 60 minutes of finishing the session makes use of that window. The muscles are primed to receive amino acids for repair. This is not complicated nutrition science; it is matching a meal to a physiological state that the practice itself has created.

Simple Before and After Practice Meal Ideas

These are practical, not prescriptive. The point is to have options ready rather than making a decision from scratch every morning. Most people find that establishing one consistent before-practice and one consistent after-practice habit removes the daily decision entirely, which reduces the friction that causes habits to collapse.

Before practice (small, 30 45 minutes prior):

Half a banana with a small spoonful of almond butter quick carbohydrate with a little fat to slow digestion. A few whole grain crackers with a thin slice of cheese similar balance of quick energy and protein. One hard-boiled egg on its own simple, protein-forward, very easy to prepare in batches the night before. A small pot of plain Greek yogurt light, high in protein, well-tolerated before movement for most people. A handful of mixed nuts and a few dried apricots or dates portable, no preparation required. Any one of these is sufficient. The goal is not a substantial meal; it is enough food to prevent energy dips and maintain focus through the session.

After practice (within 60 minutes, a proper meal if possible):

Two scrambled or poached eggs with whatever vegetables are in the refrigerator spinach, tomato, mushrooms, peppers. Ten minutes to prepare and one of the most effective post-practice meals possible. Oatmeal made with milk instead of water, with a scoop of Greek yogurt stirred in and a handful of fresh or frozen berries on top this hits protein, anti-inflammatory fruit, and complex carbohydrate in one bowl. Canned salmon or tuna with whole grain crackers, sliced cucumber, and a few cherry tomatoes no cooking, high protein, genuinely complete. A bowl of lentil or bean soup with a slice of whole grain bread anti-inflammatory legumes, good fiber, satisfying. Cottage cheese with sliced fruit and a small handful of walnuts a five-minute assembly that covers protein, healthy fat, and anti-inflammatory fruit simultaneously.

The commonality across these options is speed and protein. A meal that takes 20 minutes to prepare is less likely to happen in the post-practice window than one that takes five. Reduce the friction. Keep the ingredients accessible. Make the after-practice meal the easiest decision of the morning.

One additional note for people who practice in the afternoon or evening: the same principles apply. A small protein-containing snack before the session and a protein-containing meal within an hour after it. The timing matters more than the specific foods. The body's window of receptivity after moderate exercise does not care whether it is 7am or 5pm.

Hydration, Sleep, and the Weight Loss Triangle

These three factors water intake, sleep quality, and movement practice operate as a system. Improving one makes the others easier. Neglecting one undermines the others. For people over sixty, this triangle matters more than any specific food choice, and addressing it produces results that no dietary intervention alone can match.

Hydration.

The sensation of thirst becomes less reliable with age. Many older adults are chronically mildly dehydrated without knowing it, and mild dehydration impairs everything: joint lubrication, cortisol clearance, cognitive clarity, and the efficiency of the fat metabolism that Tai Chi supports. The kidneys require adequate water to clear the metabolic byproducts of fat oxidation. The joints require it to maintain synovial fluid. The brain requires it for the kind of focused attention that makes the forms work.

The simplest fix is to drink a glass of water before the practice session and another after it. Two glasses per day tied to an existing habit. This is not a large ask, and the effect on energy and joint comfort is often noticeable within a week. For people who struggle to drink water throughout the day, keeping a glass or small bottle visibly on the kitchen counter or the practice space as a physical reminder is more effective than trying to remember.

Caffeinated drinks coffee and tea count toward daily fluid intake and do not need to be reduced unless they are directly interfering with sleep. Alcohol is genuinely dehydrating and does impair the cortisol-clearing effect that is central to what this practice does. Reducing alcohol, particularly in the evening, has an amplifying effect on the sleep benefits of the practice that no other single change can match.

Sleep.

Adequate sleep is the most underestimated factor in weight management for older adults. During deep sleep, the body releases growth hormone, clears accumulated cortisol, and performs the cellular repair that exercise makes necessary. A practice that consistently produces better sleep as Tai Chi does through its cortisol-lowering mechanism is, in a genuine sense, a weight loss intervention operating during the hours when the practitioner is not moving at all.

The minimum effective sleep duration for metabolic health in most adults is seven hours. Under six hours, cortisol clearance is incomplete, growth hormone release is reduced, and hunger-regulating hormones shift in the direction that makes overeating more likely the following day. These are not marginal effects. They are large enough to meaningfully undercut the metabolic work the practice is doing. Protecting sleep is not optional support for the program; it is a core component of it.

Practical sleep hygiene for people doing this practice: keep a consistent wake time even on weekends this is the most effective single lever for sleep quality. Keep the bedroom cool. Avoid screens in the 45 minutes before bed. If the Tai Chi session itself is in the evening, follow it with the Closing Form held for five full breaths, then transition to something quiet. The parasympathetic activation from the practice supports sleep onset; let it do its job rather than immediately switching to something stimulating.

The triangle in practice.

A person who practices Tai Chi daily, drinks adequate water, eats enough protein, and sleeps seven to eight hours has addressed every major lever available for healthy weight management after sixty without a calorie count, without a meal plan, without adding the cognitive load of a formal diet onto an already full life. This is the sustainable version. The dramatic version produces three weeks of results and four months of backlash. The sustainable version produces 28 days of practice, a body that has changed its baseline, and habits that continue beyond the program because they feel better to maintain than to abandon.

The triangle is also self-reinforcing in the positive direction. Better sleep produces more energy for practice. More consistent practice produces lower cortisol. Lower cortisol improves sleep quality and makes food choices easier. Adequate hydration supports joint comfort in the forms. Each improvement opens the door for the next. This is what a sustainable approach to weight management after sixty actually looks like not a dramatic intervention, but a set of connected habits that improve each other over time.

Chapter 7

Strength That Lasts Beyond the Program

The 28-day program builds a practice. This chapter extends it. The five movements here are not formal Tai Chi forms. They are brief, targeted exercises designed for the gaps in the day: the kitchen, the waiting room, the moment between sitting and going somewhere.

Done consistently, they maintain and build on what the program produced. Done alongside the program, they accelerate it.

Why Muscle Matters More Than the Scale After 60

The scale measures mass. Total mass. It does not distinguish between muscle and fat, between bone and water, between a body that is getting stronger and one that is staying the same weight for the wrong reasons. This limitation is particularly significant after sixty, when the most important changes happening inside the body are often invisible to the scale.

Muscle tissue is metabolically active in a way that fat tissue is not. Every pound of muscle the body carries burns approximately six calories per day at rest. Over a year, four pounds of added functional muscle accounts for almost nine pounds of fat metabolized through resting metabolic rate alone. The scale may not move at first, because fat lost is being replaced by muscle gained. The body composition changes while the number stays the same. Then, usually around weeks six to eight of consistent practice, the scale begins to follow.

Muscle also protects. It absorbs impact before joints do. It holds the skeleton upright without the joints having to compensate. It reduces fall risk by responding quickly when balance is challenged. The frailty that many people associate with aging is not aging itself. It is the progressive loss of muscle mass that happens in the absence of consistent resistance-based movement. That loss is not inevitable. It responds to exactly the kind of slow, sustained, resistance-bearing movement this practice asks of the body.

The five movements in this chapter are not supplemental. They are the difference between a practice that maintains what you have and one that actually rebuilds what years of inactivity may have taken.

Five Micro-Movements to Stay Strong Between Sessions

Each of these takes less than two minutes. No equipment. No designated space. They can be done while waiting for a kettle to boil, standing at a bus stop, or sitting in a waiting room. The kitchen, the waiting room, the moment between sitting and going somewhere. The cumulative effect of five two-minute strength efforts distributed through the day is comparable to a single ten-minute strength session, because the muscles receive stimulation multiple times rather than all at once.

Micro-Movement 1: Wall Press

Maintains pushing strength in the arms and shoulders between full Wall Push sessions.

Starting Position:

Stand one arm's length from a smooth wall. Both palms flat on the wall at shoulder height.

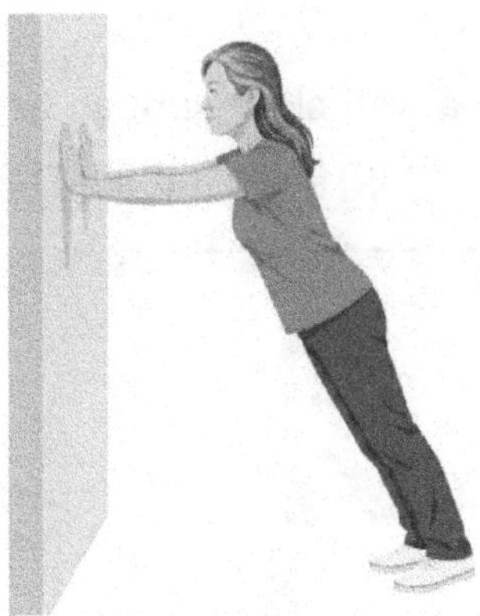

Steps:

1. Bend both elbows slowly, lowering the chest toward the wall until the elbows are at 90 degrees.

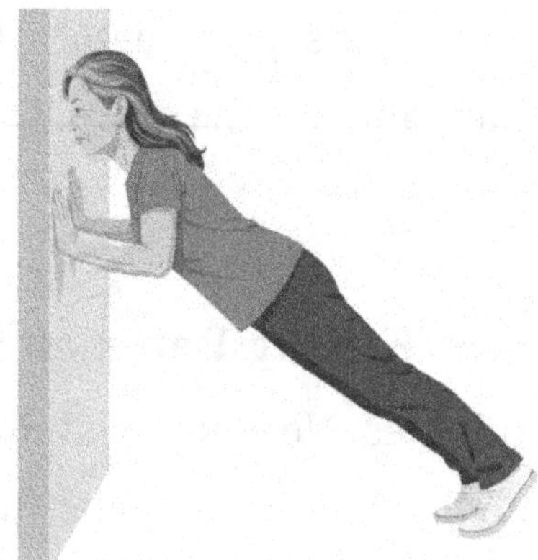

2. Press both palms into the wall and straighten the arms, returning to the starting position.

3. Complete eight slow repetitions. That is the set.

BREATHING: Inhale as you lower. Exhale as you press away.

FEEL IT: A clear engagement across the chest and back of the upper arms on the press.

SEATED MODIFICATION
Seated wall press: sit in a chair facing a wall close enough to place both palms flat on it at chest height. Same elbow bend and press movement. Eight repetitions.

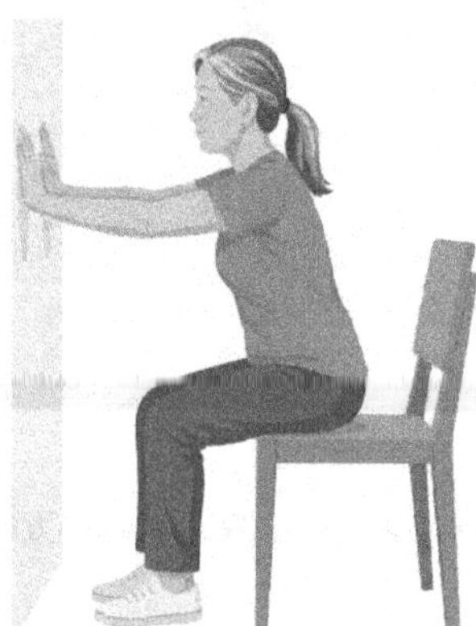

Micro-Movement 2: Standing Calf Raise

Maintains calf and ankle strength for balance and fall prevention throughout the day.

Starting Position:

Stand behind a chair with both hands resting lightly on the chair back. Feet hip-width apart.

Steps:

1. Rise slowly onto the balls of both feet, lifting the heels as high as comfortable. Keep weight even across both feet.

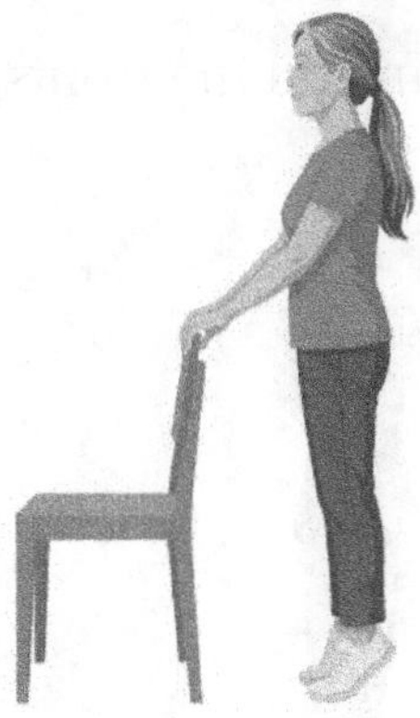

2. Hold for two counts at the top.

3. Lower the heels slowly and with full control back to the floor.

4. Complete 10 to 12 repetitions.

BREATHING: Inhale as you rise. Exhale as you lower.

FEEL IT: A clear burn in the calf muscles from repetition six onward. That is the point.

SEATED MODIFICATION

Seated calf raise: sit at the front of your chair, feet flat on the floor. Rise onto the balls of your feet, hold two counts, lower slowly. Full range, same effect. 10 to 12 repetitions.

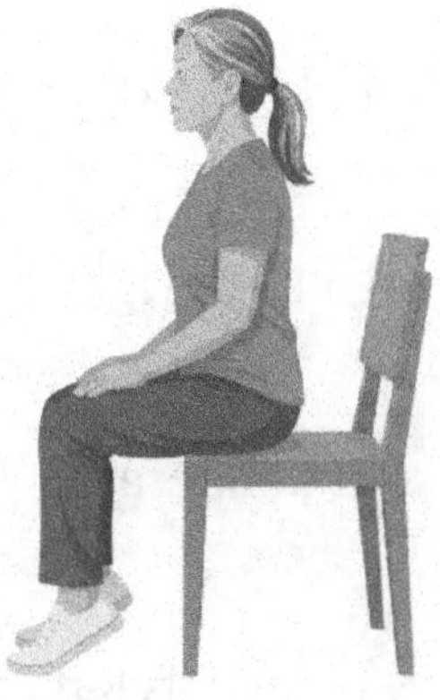

Micro-Movement 3: Hip Hinge

Strengthens the posterior chain (glutes, hamstrings, lower back) and reinforces the correct bending mechanics used throughout daily life.

Starting Position:

Stand with feet hip-width apart, hands resting on the fronts of the thighs.

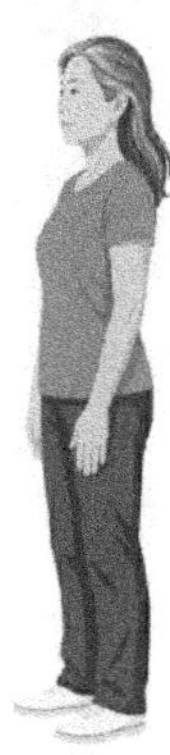

Steps:

1. Push both hips backward as you hinge forward from the hips, not the waist. Let the hands slide down the thighs as the torso tips forward. Spine stays long, not rounded.

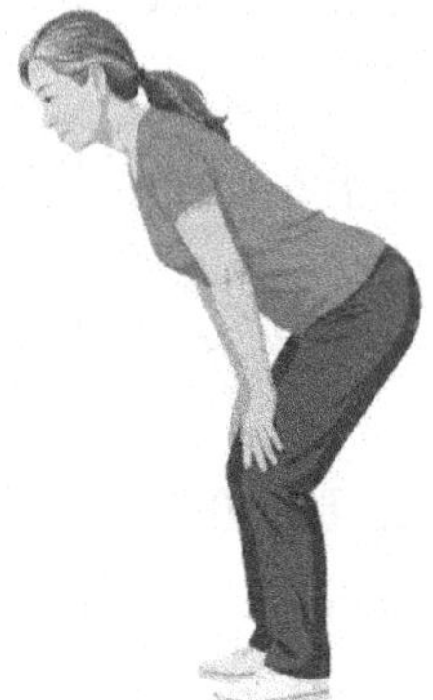

2. Pause when the torso reaches roughly 45 degrees from upright. Feel the stretch in the backs of the thighs.

3. Drive the hips forward and return to upright by squeezing the glutes. Do not pull up with the lower back.

4. Complete 10 repetitions, slow and deliberate.

BREATHING: Inhale as you hinge forward. Exhale as you drive back to upright.

FEEL IT: A stretch in the hamstrings on the way down, a clear glute engagement on the drive back up.

SEATED MODIFICATION
From your chair, lean forward from the hips with a long flat spine, then press through the feet and stand. That is a seated-to-standing hip hinge. The same muscles in the same pattern. 10 repetitions.

Micro-Movement 4: Doorframe Row

Strengthens the upper back and postural muscles that prevent the forward shoulder rounding common in people who sit for extended periods.

Starting Position:

Stand in a doorframe with both hands gripping the frame at shoulder height, one hand on each side. Step your feet close enough to the frame so your arms are extended with a slight lean back.

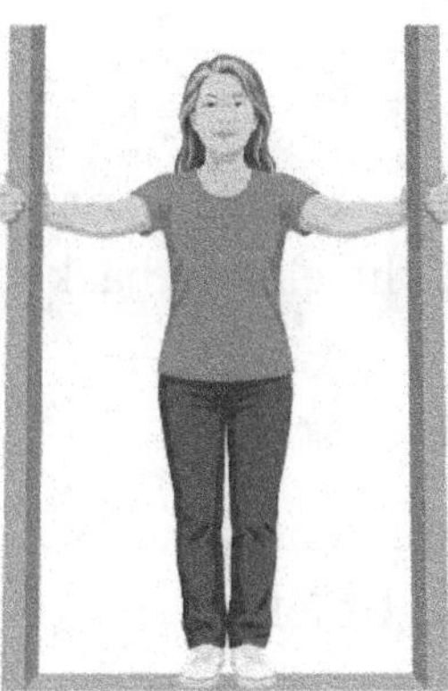

Steps:

1. Pull both elbows back, drawing your chest toward the doorframe. Keep the elbows close to the body.

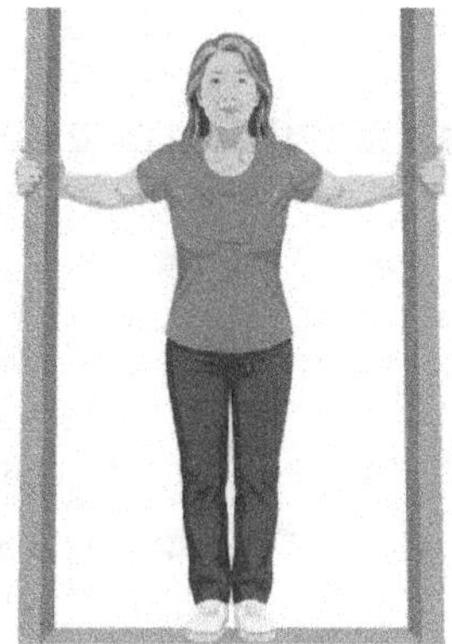

2. Pause when the chest reaches the frame or as far as comfortable.

3. Extend both arms back to the starting position under control.

4. Complete eight to 10 repetitions.

BREATHING: Exhale as you pull. Inhale as you extend.

FEEL IT: A clear engagement across the upper back and between the shoulder blades on the pull.

SEATED MODIFICATION

Loop a towel around a fixed door handle. Sit in a chair facing the door, holding both ends of the towel. Lean back slightly and pull the elbows back toward your hips. Same upper back muscles. Eight to 10 repetitions.

Micro-Movement 5: Lateral Weight Shift

Maintains the balance mechanics and hip stabilizers trained in Cloud Hands, reinforcing fall prevention outside of practice sessions.

Starting Position:

Stand near a wall or chair back for balance reference. Feet slightly wider than shoulder-width. Hands at your sides or lightly touching the support.

Steps:

1. Shift your weight slowly onto your left foot, feeling the floor through the whole left foot. Let the right heel lift slightly.

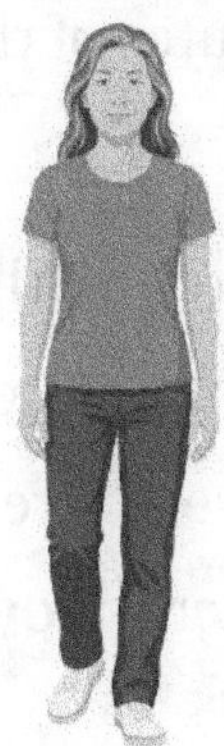

2. Hold for three counts. Feel the hip stabilizers engage on the left side.

3. Shift slowly to the right. Hold three counts.

4. Complete 10 full shifts, five each side. Slow and deliberate the whole way through.

BREATHING: Breathe naturally. One full breath per shift.

FEEL IT: A quiet but definite engagement in the outer hip on the weight-bearing side. This is the same mechanism that prevents sideways stumbles.

SEATED MODIFICATION
Seated lateral weight shift: sit at the front of your chair and shift your weight slightly left so the left sit-bone presses down more than the right. Hold three counts. Shift right. Same hip stabilizers, supported by the seat. 10 shifts.

Balance, Stability, and Joint Protection

The forms in Chapter Four replicate the exact mechanics the body uses every day in ways most people have stopped practicing. Cloud Hands trains the lateral weight shift that keeps you stable when you reach across a table. Parting the Wild Horse's Mane trains the stepping mechanics that protect the hip when walking on uneven ground. The Closing Form trains the controlled deceleration that prevents a stumble from becoming a fall.

Balance is not a fixed capacity. It degrades with disuse and improves with practice. The Tai Chi neutral stance is itself a balance exercise, because it requires constant small adjustments to stay upright on soft, ready feet. Ten minutes of this daily is more effective balance training than most people have had in years.

Joint protection comes from the muscles around the joint, not from the joint structure itself. Strong quadriceps protect the knee. Strong glutes protect the hip. A strong and mobile shoulder girdle protects the rotator cuff. Every Strength Builder in this chapter targets one of these protective muscle groups. The five micro-movements maintain that protection between formal sessions.

Feeling Younger on Your Feet

This phrase is in the book's subtitle, and it deserves a plain account of what it actually refers to. Not a vague sense of vitality. Something specific.

The feeling is proprioceptive confidence. Proprioception is the body's internal sense of its own position in space. It tells you where your foot is without looking. It is the mechanism that prevents a stumble on an uneven sidewalk from becoming a fall, because the body corrects before the brain has time to register the problem. Proprioception declines with age, and it is one of the primary contributors to fall risk after sixty. It also responds directly and quickly to the kind of practice in this book.

When people say they feel younger after consistent Tai Chi practice, they are usually describing this: moving through the world with more ease and less hesitation. Getting up from a chair without thinking about it. Walking down a step without pausing. Turning quickly without grabbing something. The difference between living in the body with confidence and living in it with caution. That is what the practice gives back.

Chapter 8

After Day 28

The program is finished. Before you decide what happens next, read this chapter. It will help you interpret what you experienced over the past 28 days and give you a clear picture of the options available from here.

Reading Your Results Honestly

There is no single correct outcome for a 28-day Tai Chi program. The range of genuine results is wide, and all of it is real. What matters is understanding what you are actually measuring and what the measurements mean.

If your balance improved noticeably by Day 28, that is a physiological change. The stabilizing muscles around your ankles and hips got stronger. The proprioceptive pathways were stimulated daily. The nervous system built new balance patterns. These changes are structural. They do not disappear when the program ends, because they are not the result of medication or equipment. They are built into the body. A person who holds a single-leg balance for 20 seconds on Day 28 when they could barely manage 5 on assessment day has not reached a temporary state. They have changed the underlying architecture.

If your morning stiffness eased, that is the synovial fluid effect working. Joints that receive daily movement produce more lubricating fluid than joints that do not. This is also a structural change, and it is also cumulative. It will continue to improve with continued practice. The people who report the most dramatic joint improvements are usually those who reach the three-month mark of consistent practice, not the four-week mark. The 28 days started something. The next two months complete it.

If your energy improved, your sleep changed, or something in how you carry yourself shifted, those are the cortisol and cardiovascular effects. They are genuine and they are dose-dependent: more consistent practice produces larger effects over time. Some people describe a steadier quality to their mornings. Some describe a reduction in the afternoon energy drop that had become normal. Some describe sleeping through the night for the first time in years. These are not placebo effects. They are measurable hormonal changes that happen to people who practice in the way this program prescribes.

If the scale did not move much, that may mean several things. It may mean that fat loss and muscle gain happened simultaneously and offset each other. It may mean that the first month of any new practice produces more preparatory change than visible change. It may mean that food patterns are working against the metabolic effects of the practice. Chapter Six addresses this directly. The scale is the last indicator to trust and the least informative of the set. What did your clothes do? What did your balance do? What did your morning feel like at Day 28 compared to Day 1?

Whatever happened over the past 28 days, be honest with it. Don't minimize the real changes because they weren't dramatic. Don't manufacture improvements that aren't there. Work with what is actually true, because the decisions below depend on an accurate reading.

What to Do If Progress Stalled

If you completed all 28 days and feel that little changed, there are four common reasons. One of them is almost certainly the explanation.

Inconsistent practice.

The compounding effects described in Chapter Two require daily or near-daily practice to build. A program where seven of the 28 sessions were skipped is a different physiological intervention than a complete one. If this was the case, a second 28-day attempt with higher attendance will produce different results. The attendance does not need to be perfect. It needs to be consistent. Five out of seven days sustains the cortisol regulation and muscle adaptation effects. Three out of seven does not.

Insufficient sleep.

If you slept under six hours consistently during the program, the cortisol clearance and growth hormone release that drive the body composition changes did not happen at full capacity. This is not a minor variable. Sleep is where the adaptation occurs. The practice creates the stimulus and sleep is where the body responds to it. Protecting sleep during a second attempt, even if the change required is going to bed 45 minutes earlier, will change the outcome more than any modification to the practice itself.

Food patterns working against the practice.

Chronic undereating reduces muscle protein synthesis and signals the body to protect stored fat. Chronic overconsumption of refined carbohydrates sustains the insulin resistance that the practice is trying to reverse. Neither of these is a judgment. Both are information. The adjustments in Chapter Six are specific and manageable, and making them for a second 28-day round will produce a different metabolic outcome than the first.

Insufficient intensity progression.

The program is designed to progress week by week, with rep counts and session lengths increasing at each stage. If the Week Four sessions felt no harder than Week One, the progression may not have been applied fully. Week Three and Four should be perceptibly more demanding. If they were not, adding two more reps to each exercise and extending the form sequences in a second round will address this.

If you identify your reason, you have your adjustment. A second attempt with the specific variable changed will demonstrate whether that variable was the limiting factor. Most people who do a second round of the program with one specific adjustment see the difference they were looking for the first time.

How to Keep Going Without Starting Over

Not everyone wants to repeat the program. Not everyone needs to. There are two clean options.

Option A: Repeat the program.

Run the 28-day program again from Day 1. This works particularly well if Week One was rough and you want a cleaner experience of the full arc. The movements are familiar now. The early sessions will feel different when the forms are not being learned simultaneously. Most people who run the program a second time find it qualitatively different, because the learning load is gone and the practice itself can be felt more clearly. The physical experience of Cloud Hands on Day 8 of a second run is not the same as Cloud Hands on Day 8 of the first run. The body knows what it is doing.

Option B: Use Chapter Four as a daily library.

Build your own daily practice from the seven forms and four Strength Builders in Chapter Four. Choose what to include based on how the body feels that day. A minimum practice on a low-energy day might be Cloud Hands, Wave Hands Like Clouds, and the Closing Form. A full practice might be all seven forms, two Strength Builders, and the warm-up sequence. The program's job was to teach you the forms. Your job now is to use them in whatever combination serves the morning you have.

Either option maintains the practice. The only wrong choice is stopping entirely because the program ended. The program was not the goal. The habit was the goal. Programs end. Habits don't need to.

Building a Practice That Lasts Beyond the Book

A sustainable long-term practice has three characteristics. It is short enough to be done on any day, including bad ones. It is flexible enough to adapt to the body's state on a given morning. And it ends with something that feels worth doing again tomorrow.

The Closing Form is in the program for this third reason. It is not just a cool-down. It is a signal to the nervous system and to the practicing mind that the session is complete, that something happened, and that it will happen again. Every session that ends with the Closing Form is a session that contains a natural stopping point rather than just stopping. Over time, the Closing Form becomes associated with the particular feeling that follows practice, and that association is what makes people return to it even on days when they would rather not.

Long-term Tai Chi practice does not look like the 28-day program. It looks like ten minutes most mornings, sometimes fifteen, occasionally five, practiced with the same attention whether the body is willing or not. It looks like the warm-up sequence done on rest days when the full practice is not possible. It looks like one of the micro-movements from Chapter Seven done in the kitchen while something is heating. It looks like the Foundational Breathing Practice used before a difficult conversation.

The practice expands to fill available time and contracts to fit constrained time. This is its great advantage over more elaborate exercise formats, which require a minimum time commitment to be worth doing and therefore are not done on the days that minimum cannot be met. A Tai Chi practice can be one breathing sequence and the Closing Form on the worst possible morning. It is still a practice. The nervous system still received the signal. The habit is still intact.

The practice is not bounded by the book or the program. It is bounded by the body you have and the ten minutes you are willing to give it. Both of those things are, and have always been, enough.

Did You Find This Book Quite Helpful?

If it did, then that's worth something and deserves a place on Amazon.

A short review on Amazon takes two minutes and costs nothing. But for an independent author with no marketing budget, it means everything. It is how the next reader finds this book. It is how a daughter finds the right gift for her aging mother and father. It is how this work continues to reach the people it was made for.

Search ***Tai Chi for Weight Loss by Jing Weston*** on Amazon. One or two honest sentences is all it takes.

Thank you for reading. It was an honor to take this trip with you.

Conclusion

Something changes when a person who was not moving starts moving. Not just in the body, but in the relationship with the body.

What This Practice Gives Back

After sixty, the body requires things from exercise that most popular exercise formats are not designed to provide. It needs movement that lubricates joints rather than grinding them. It needs breathe work that lowers cortisol rather than spiking it. It needs strength training that builds functional capacity rather than exhausting it. It needs practices short enough to be done consistently and complete enough to produce real change.

Tai Chi provides all of these things in ten minutes, in a living room, with no equipment. This is not a coincidence. It is the product of centuries of refinement by people who understood that the body at every age responds to different demands differently, and who developed a movement practice specifically calibrated to work with the aging body rather than against it.

What the practice gives back is not the body of a younger person. It gives back a better relationship with the body you currently have. More trust in it. More confidence moving through the world in it. More ease in the ordinary moments that most people take for granted until they start to cost something. Getting up from a chair without thinking about it. Crossing a room without pausing at the threshold. Walking down a step without bracing for it. These are small things and they are enormous things, depending on whether or not you still have them.

The practice restores some of what time takes. Not all of it. But more than most people expect, and consistently enough to be reliable.

Finishing a Program and Starting a Habit

The 28-day program was a container for learning. Every form is now in the body. The breath sequence is familiar. The warm-up sequence is yours. The Closing Form is yours. These are not things that live in this book. They live in you now, in the physical memory of having done them for 28 consecutive days.

Finishing the program is not the same as building the habit. The habit is built by continuing. Not heroically, not at great cost, but consistently. The same ten minutes tomorrow morning that there was today. And the next day. And the day after that.

This is how the compounding effects described in Chapter Two actually work. They are not produced by 28 days of practice. They are produced by 90 days, 180 days, a year. The 28-day program is not the destination. It is the beginning of a sufficient relationship with movement to sustain the next six months of practice, which produces the next round of physical change, which makes the following year easier. The people who get the most from this practice are not the ones who start with the most enthusiasm. They are the ones who are still at it in month six.

Final Word from Jing

The people I have worked with who stayed with this practice the longest were not the ones who started with the most discipline. They were the ones who started with enough curiosity to keep going when the discipline ran out.

Somewhere around Day 12 or Day 15, something usually shifts. The movement stops feeling like an instruction and starts feeling like something the body already knows. The breath coordinates itself without counting. The transition from one form to the next begins to feel like one thing rather than two. When that happens, you are not following the practice anymore. You are practicing. That distinction matters more than it sounds.

I have watched people arrive at that moment after two weeks, and I have watched others arrive at it after two months. The timeline is individual. What is not individual is the moment itself. It happens for everyone who stays with it long enough.

That is where I will leave you. The forms are in the book if you need them. The program is there if you want to run it again. But the practice, the actual thing that produces the changes this book describes, is already yours.

Go practice.

About the Author

Jing Weston has practiced Tai Chi for more than two decades and has spent most of that time working with older adults, people managing chronic conditions, and beginners who came to movement late and found it transformed how they lived. He began with group classes at a community center and eventually worked one-on-one with people whose physical constraints required a more individualized approach: patients recovering from joint replacements, people with severe balance deficits, adults in their eighties who had been sedentary for years and wanted to change that.

His teaching approach is grounded in a single conviction: that the body at any age responds to appropriate, consistent movement. Not to dramatic intervention. Not to punishment. To the kind of slow, deliberate, breath-coordinated practice that Tai Chi represents at its core. He has seen this conviction validated too many times to hold it lightly.

He holds decades of attention to how older bodies move, what helps them, and what does not. This book is an attempt to make that attention available to people who cannot be in the same room with him.

He lives simply and practices every morning, usually before the day has fully started.

www.ingramcontent.com/pod-product-compliance
Lightning Source LLC
Chambersburg PA
CBHW080339030726
47594CB00012B/4084